THE HEAVENS ARE ALL BLUE

Dr Finbar Lennon is a medical graduate of University College Dublin (UCD). He trained in Dublin, London and Edmonton. He was appointed a consultant general surgeon in Our Lady of Lourdes Hospital in Drogheda in 1982. Since his retirement in 2012, he has taught undergraduate medical students in the Mater Hospital in Dublin. He was recently appointed an adjunct Associate Professor in Clinical Surgery in UCD.

Dr Kate McGarry was an honours medical graduate of UCD. She was awarded the Bellingham Gold Medal in Clinical Medicine in St Vincent's Hospital in 1972 where she did her early postgraduate training. Her later training took place in the Hammersmith and Great Ormond Street hospitals in London and in the Clinical Pharmacology Department in the Royal College of Surgeons in Ireland. She was appointed a Clinical Cardiology Fellow in University Hospital, Edmonton in Canada before returning to Ireland in 1983 to take up a post as a consultant physician in Our Lady's Hospital in Navan. During her tenure there, she was instrumental in developing its cardiology services. She became a Fellow of the Royal College of Physicians in Ireland (RCPI) in 1985 and served as an elected member of its council for 25 years. She was appointed President of the Irish Heart Foundation in 2015. She died in January 2018. In October 2019, the RCPI in honouring her memory created a prestigious new award, the Dr Kate McGarry prize, to be awarded annually to doctors in training posts.

Dr FINBAR LENNON and
Dr KATE McGARRY

The
Heavens
are all
Blue

HACHETTE
BOOKS
IRELAND

First published in Ireland in 2020 by
HACHETTE BOOKS IRELAND

1

Cataloguing in Publication Data is available from the British Library

ISBN 978 1 5293 6238 1

Typeset in Bembo Book MT Std by Bookends Publishing Services, Dublin

Printed and bound in Great Britain by Clays Ltd, Elcograf, S.p.A

Hachette Books Ireland policy is to use papers that are natural, renewable and recyclable
products and made from wood grown in sustainable forests. The logging and manufacturing
processes are expected to conform to the environmental regulations of the country of origin.

Hachette Books Ireland
8 Castlecourt Centre
Castleknock
Dublin 15, Ireland

A division of Hachette UK Ltd
Carmelite House, 50 Victoria Embankment, EC4Y 0DZ

www.hachettebooksireland.ie

For Ruth

Dedicated to our four wonderful children David, Ruth, Peter and Stephen, our four grandchildren Finn, Harry, Maisie and Teddy and to the four McGarry sibs, Patricia, Michael, Joan and Paul.

CONTENTS

PROLOGUE

The headstone will crack and splinter,
The names and dates will fade,
The bones beneath will lose their moorings;
When the grandchildren call in 50 years,
The only link between us
Will be what is written now.

Connemara, July 2017
I have decided to write a book about my personal experience
with cancer, as a doctor who becomes a patient. At the time
of my diagnosis a physician friend of mine said I would find
'silver linings' in this phase of my life. Perhaps if people survive
cancer they can look back and develop new perspectives on
their lives and see the experience as somewhat enriching.

But what about me? I am not likely to get better, so what
'silver linings' can I expect? Maybe when I finish this book I
will have some new message that will help my fellow patients,
or maybe not. And so, on a rainy day in Connemara, I have
started to write this story, not knowing what the end chapter

will be. Last Friday we attended the burial of the ashes of a dear friend at the beautiful Renvyle cemetery in Cashleen. It reminded me that death will find us whoever and wherever we are.

If you last long enough, it's the lungs that kill you in the end. Gasping for breath is not worth fighting for, and too much medicine brings you there. Even the 'darling Zimos', as she fondly called the reliable sleeping pills she took every night, did not work in her final months. The heavy-duty artillery infusions were needed to dull the senses and ease her passage. This is a story about an ending. The principals are all real people. The storyline is commonplace. It is a tragedy for those involved, but not remarkable in itself. People die all the time and don't receive any special mention. Life and death go hand in hand, and each life is forgotten over time. The span of it, short or long, is immaterial. Sometimes an individual's case is reported in dispatches. Perhaps they were someone famous, a leader or a follower who made a difference. In this case, the person in question was the love of my life.

As far back as I can remember, everybody called her Kate, but she was always Kathleen to me, or Mum within our own family, and so it remained even after the children left home. The original intention was for her to write a memoir detailing her experience of living and coping with cancer. She recorded in diary form her personal observations on her illness and treatment. She wrote all of these excerpts on her fading life in flowing handwriting with gradually diminishing and then no spaces between the words. She was in a hurry. There were things she wanted to say for, and about, herself and her family. She was the main character in the story. She did not want to leave the reader in any doubt about her knowledge of her illness, her emotions or the importance of the family bonds and solidarity that sustained her. She packed a lot of information into short segments of prose and often in random order. Some of it was repetitive, for effect, but all was part of the same canvas, spread over separate pages of her two working diaries, ready to be placed in order and given some form by the loving, discerning hand of one she trusted to recount her story of darkness and light. I hope this narrative will also reveal a life of service and virtue.

Before Kathleen died, I promised I would write 'the book' for her. I was an important character in her story and she wanted me to contribute to it equally, to make it into a joint enterprise. And so it became our book.

'Of course, you know I won't be a ghost writer,' I said jokingly to her. 'I will appear in the book from time to time (a lot of the time), trying to make an impression!'

'That's OK,' she replied. 'I will be happy as long as you are writing for me and about us.'

I spent six months poring over her diaries and notebooks, where she had outlined her medical history and her recollections and commentary about her illness and its impact on her over its 18-month duration. I read a number of recent medical memoirs and books on how to write memoirs. At the end of August 2018, I went on one of my regular bus trips to Dublin, attended Mass in Berkeley Road Church beside the Mater Hospital, had breakfast in the hospital canteen and called by the student teaching centre to arrange my bedside tutorials for the coming term. I then walked down to Parnell Square and called in to the Irish Writers Centre, of which I had recently become a member, and booked onto a creative writing course for that autumn, before having lunch with two of my sisters. On the afternoon bus home, I decided to browse Google for tips on how to write a memoir. The first advice I found was from the doyenne of New York publishing, Jane Friedman, and it was a reality check that hurt. For many sound reasons, all evidence based, she implied that I, like the majority of other first-time writers, could not do it and should not even try – and this struck an unwelcome chord in my medical brain. I opened the bag I had with me and took out Christopher Hitchens' memoir, *Mortality*, and read the first three chapters once again. I could never write like him! His book is touted as one of the best, and only the best are published. Suddenly deflated and wondering what to do next, I contemplated my dilemma. After considered reflection, I decided to ignore Friedman's warnings and Hitchens' impossibly high bar for the moment. I knew I needed to get on with it now, as Kathleen would have said, and of course it would be all about her.

We were two successful doctors who had spent 30 years in hospital practice as specialty consultants, she in general medicine and me in surgery, and we were acknowledged as competent in our respective areas of practice. I could have said 'experts' and our peers would not have demurred! The management and care of patients with cancer was a significant part of our clinical work. She was brighter than me, I'm happy to acknowledge, and a high achiever from her early student days; during her professional working life, she was invited to take on many vocational and representative roles by her professional college and the Minister for Health of the day. In short, she was a star and acknowledged as such by all her contemporaries.

When Kathleen commenced her consultant practice in Ireland in the 1980s, the sick patients who depended on her had to rely on her knowledge and wits for their survival. Every hospital in the country in that era admitted emergency cases, but few had the range of diagnostic and treatment technology needed to provide a consistent standard of care for all acute conditions. The decision to treat onsite or transfer was often a risky and difficult call that the primary clinician had to make alone. When she handed on the baton after 30 years at Our Lady's Hospital in Navan, most of the essential diagnostic technological equipment was finally available onsite there. Unfortunately, when it came to her turn and she became ill, those advances and the many new developments in medical treatment that had occurred during her professional life were not sufficient to come to her aid, and so ultimately she too had to put her trust in the knowledge and wits of her peers.

A few months after Kathleen's death in January 2018, a copy of *Cancer Professional*, an Irish quarterly specialist cancer journal, arrived in the post, along with a few late condolence letters and Mass cards. The title of an article highlighted on its front cover caught my eye: 'Cancer of unknown primary origin (CUP)'. Since this was the label Kathleen's cancer had been given, I read the piece with mixed feelings and mainly out of a sense of duty to her. Often described as a 'forgotten' cancer, CUP accounts for less than 3 per cent of all cancers and is one where the patient's clinical course is one of complete uncertainty. It is a devastating diagnosis because it presents with disease that has already spread, with no identifiable primary site. There is no standard management strategy and the treatment is empirical (i.e. hit-and-miss). The diagnostic work-up involves multiple investigations and the best that can be achieved is a reasonable conjecture as to the tissue of origin.

Now that Kathleen is gone, I am the only one who can write and complete her memoir. The one qualification I have is that I am old enough to write a love story – and while that is only part of the multi-layered 'documentary' of her life, it provides the energy and imagination to see this through. Sit down, find pen and paper and start writing – it sounds easy. Perhaps it is easy for a creative writer, which I will have to become if I am to finish this book. First, I have to lay out the facts in sentences and paragraphs, but more importantly, choose the words and punctuation to create a rounded picture. Then I have to change, chop and discard until the essential elements are visible and discernible. I am also aware that I must part with convention and compose a book with two active participating authors.

I know where to start but it is difficult to know what to say. Like so many others before us, ours was a love story cut short, seemingly at random, by an act of God (or is that attribution of blame fair?). Kathleen's cancer struck relatively late in her natural life cycle and near the end of her professional career in medicine. Retirement and our children's emerging family formations were beckoning, and we were looking forward to more time spent together and new milestones in the years ahead. But, having read a number of recently published memoirs about death from cancer, I wondered what our experiences had to add to the mix that was different and compelling.

Then I realised hers was a case of an unusual cancer in an uncommon patient and that, as such, it's a story that has not been told before. Our combined medical experience and perspectives might add a new twist to an account of an unpredictable illness, where the doctor is taking the medicine instead of prescribing it. The story of a doctor trying to influence her own life's final journey rather than that of one of her patients perhaps brings a new dimension in itself. In the creative writing class, we were told that the strength of memoir lies in its ability to evoke an emotional response in the reader – and there, too, I hope I can make an impression.

Paul Kalanithi, a brilliant neurosurgeon and humanitarian whose life was cut short by a devastating cancer, had just enough time to write most of his memoir, *When Breath Becomes Air*; his wife, also a medical consultant, completed it for him, as I hope now to do for Kathleen. It strikes me that Paul and Kathleen were kindred spirits in many ways. Like him, she wanted to tell her own story; both he and she had medical spouses who also spent their working lives manning the front lines. The absence of the work–life balance and its harmful impact on professional lives was not recognised until recent years. Paul did not live long enough to see its folly, but when she became a consultant, Kathleen did attempt to address the problem on behalf of the junior trainee doctors and the next generation of medical specialists. Paul's crusade in medicine was an unforgiving mission where the stakes were always high. It was to battle death with his hands, his mind and his voice as a surgeon and companion of his patients and then, in the midst of his final formation, to 'face the music' himself. Kathleen's mission, to which she devoted so much of her energy and determination as a specialty doctor, was to reduce the incidence of early preventable cardiovascular mortality, but she had more space and time to do so. She was self-effacing, low-key; she went about her mission and vocation with the minimum of fuss or drama. Much of her work was done when the cancer struck, and even then, she was determined to reach certain important milestones, professionally and most of all personally, before her illness had its final say. Death had to wait until she was ready!

When I took on the mantle of telling her story, I was at a loss as to whether I was up to the task. I'd always had an interest in writing and in things literary; I had the time and had made the commitment. That was the easy part of the equation. But my frame of mind and the approach I took had to be right. My emotional state created some difficulty because it varied from day to day. Although I could not always control my grief, at least I was aware of its presence. The emotional man does not seek attention but cannot hide, because his handkerchief, wet with tears, is always visible. I had to ensure my temperament did not compromise the essential objectivity of the work; that the clean lines of the story are not muddied by self-pity and a loss of perspective on my part. On that score I hope I can deliver.

Doctors do develop and retain certain narration skills due to the nature of their work. Although I have no experience of writing a memoir, I can write an essay and compose a scientific paper. Developing that competency was part of my professional training and formation. As I was not pursuing an academic career, I did not need to maintain it once my practice was established, but the skillset was already there. Kathleen worked in an academic context at certain times in her career and so had all these competencies and more, but she was also committed to telling the tale of her illness in a stark and frank way and, most importantly, with a human touch. In the short time she had, she managed to do that with insight and clarity.

And so it is Kathleen's words that will tell the essential story of her illness, while mine, dependent as I am on the emotional voice pushing the pen, will recount how we lived and coped together through the pain and anguish it caused. I cannot change or edit her recorded words but I can try to place them to best reflect her primary intent. I will travel a distance every day and stop abruptly because the tank is empty; I will start again another day and must simply go where the story takes me. A torrent of words may flow or just a trickle. I will not rest until the large and small writ is recorded, and each of these may take as long to compose and yet be all in vain. All I know is that I am travelling with the person I love and I will not stop until the work is done. I know I will redraft this paragraph at least ten times and yet the readers will pass over it in the blink of an eye. The number of words should not matter but it does for the novice, who measures worth in volume and fails to see the associated risk, that more is often less.

My task is to be an honest and faithful storyteller and, by offering a commentary from each of us, to give an insight into our dual perspectives and imbue the tale with a sense of our churning emotions. But just describing what happened is not enough – to really tell Kathleen's story, I have to go back to the beginning.

PART ONE

1

BEGINNINGS

2008
Wow! You're 60!
To the man I met in the
Bicycle Shed in 1966
Love xx, Mum

We met in the bicycle shed on the Belfield campus of University College Dublin (UCD) in 1966, and got to know each other on the rides to and from classes. I was 18; Kathleen was 17. Our first encounter occurred after class early in the first term as we were about to set off home. She was bending down to remove her bicycle from the cycle rack.

'Are you having trouble unlocking your bike?'

She turned to me, smiled and raised her eyebrows. 'What do you think?' she said, as she attempted to prise the bike loose. She was wearing glasses, which made her look thoughtful and serious – until she laughed, when it all fell apart.

I freed her bike and introduced myself.

'Where are you going?' she asked.

'To Mount Merrion.'

'So am I,' she replied and laughed again.

It was the laugh that captured me. Off we went together and I don't recall there was much conversation as we struggled up North Avenue, neither of us wanting to dismount and lose momentum. By the time we reached the summit, we had discovered we were both doing Medicine. I could not believe my luck when she reached her home on South Avenue and I realised she was living very close to me. I did not tell her then because I needed time to modify my rural manners and customs: it was a new experience for me to be involved with 'the opposite sex', and I had to adjust my emotional compass in order to survive the close encounters to come.

I was a slow learner and I was shy and did not immediately capitalise on my good fortune. So, instead of riding up and down to college and getting to know her, I decided I would avoid her for some weeks, which would be easy as there were alternative routes to Belfield and the pre-medical class was very big. However, I did not factor into my calculations that she was looking out for me, and we soon met again and got into a cycling routine together. It felt easy to talk about class work and family and gradually we learned more about both our family histories.

By that stage I had worked out a few questions to ask.

'How come you decided to do Medicine?'

'Well,' she said, 'I did not know what to do, so I did a

psychology test and was told Medicine was a good choice for me. What about you?'

'Oh, my dad is a doctor, and the Lennons always had a fair share of doctors, nurses or priests!'

She thought that was hilarious and started to laugh. I was taken aback and decided not to divulge much more about myself for the moment. I thought she was a very good-looking girl but I could only see her moving profile on a bicycle and it was a while before I could observe and study her face and features up close. But when the chance came to stare unnoticed, she looked lovely, which is the country equivalent of beautiful. It was her face and her facial expressions that I most remember. I saw the full picture instantly and I fell for her from the beginning.

I was never good on detail. Throughout our life together, I had moments of acute anxiety when I wondered, if she got lost, would I be able to give the police a description of her? I could give some idea of her height and shape, but after that it was a guess. What about the colour of her eyes and her hair? Well, her hair was always changing from long to short and, by her mid-forties onwards, from one colour tint to another. I could never remember what she was wearing from one day to the next or the colour code of her outfits – dress or slacks; flat shoes or heels; size and shape of handbag. That was no problem at the beginning. I made a point of complimenting her on her hairstyle and her clothes every time we met.

She told me a bit about herself and where she went to school and I filled her in some more on my own family. She lived at home with her parents and four sibs and I lived nearby, with a loving, caring aunt who kept my parents in Edenderry updated on my vocational and social activities. I was comfortable when she was talking, as her facial expression was easy and relaxed, but when she was listening, she focused on me with an intent gaze as if I was an oracle, which made me feel more than a little self-conscious!

After about 50 miles of cycling together to test the waters, I was ready to ask her out on a date.

'Would you like to go to the pictures?'

'You mean the films?' she said with a mischievous smile as she readily agreed.

The venue was the local cinema, within walking distance of her home, so it felt like a safe assignation and no pressure for a young man from rural Ireland with little experience of the world of dating. I walked up to her house to collect her and pressed the bell of number 47. Her mother answered and had a warm welcome for me. She knew my name and had a lovely relaxed smile like her daughter; from the moment I saw her, I knew we would get on well with each other. For her part, she seemed to take an instant liking to me too, in spite of my reserve and rarefied country manners. She made a bit of a fuss about me before Kathleen and I left to walk hand in hand to the Stella.

I bought the tickets and the popcorn and we settled into

our seats for the show. There was no need – or time – to talk because we were both busy munching. We tilted our heads to each other and our glasses clinked! She started to laugh and that broke the spell. I had to wait for another opportunity to make a meaningful advance. Kissing was a problem, as we were both short-sighted and each wore large spectacles that prevented lip contact unless one set of specs was removed. I eventually worked that out by removing hers.

Neither of us was much into passion at the time. I was naïve and unworldly because of my sheltered background in a remote part of County Offaly, and although she was much more familiar with the business of going on dates, Kathleen had little interest in getting into anything too involved at this stage in her life. She need not have worried. She was as safe as houses with me! Hence our early trysts were largely platonic, and this suited both of us, as we had a lot to learn. Besides, there was not much time for romance in the pre-med year. Our days were filled with lectures and study. As only half the class would progress to the first medical year proper, my prospects of prolonging our relationship depended on both of us passing the year-end exam and finishing in the top half of the class. That did not present a problem for her! And, fortunately, I managed it too.

The bike rides continued but became less predictable and less frequent than before, and so I used the house phone as a lifeline to keep in touch – though it was a tricky business to manage. The custom in her house was that the telephone was reserved for urgent family business and not used for intimate conversations, not least because it was located in the busiest section of the house, just inside the front door. It had not yet found its way to the bedroom! When the phone rang, it drew the whole household towards its melodic tones, and all ears would be tuned as the handset was lifted and the mystery caller identified. Whenever I phoned, Kathleen usually answered, perhaps because she had a sixth sense or was standing in the vicinity, waiting for a call from any number of 'suspects'! The exchange between us had to be brief, its only purpose being to arrange a discreet meeting place to advance our stuttering love affair, which more than once came close to stalling altogether. The meeting places never turned out to be discreet, however, and were often the front sitting rooms of her house or my aunt's house, while the 'elixir' to stimulate a cosy chat would be tea and buns.

Our first formal date was an outing to Wynn's Hotel in the city centre for an early-bird five-course dinner in its famous dining room – for 17 shillings and 6 pence each – followed by a night at the movies in the Cinerama cinema in Talbot Street. Kathleen was wearing a bright blouse with a tied bow at the neck. She had long, shiny dark-brown hair that fell over her shoulders. She was wearing a short skirt to show off her legs, which were on display not only to please and tease me but, I suspect, also for general release on the city streets that evening! Her characteristic flighty sense of fun and excitement attracted and unnerved me. I was, for a long time, more interested in poetry than passion, and she was determined to change all that!

Before we had left her house that evening to catch a bus, she had begun to rummage in her handbag, trying to find something. 'Got them!' she finally exclaimed, as she fished out her keys – and then hid them safely again in the bag. It was a scene that would be repeated countless times throughout her life. She was wearing contact lenses for the night, though she had her 'rescue specs' in the handbag in case. I smiled to myself, as it would make kissing easier, if it came to that.

She did most of the talking on the bus. She asked a lot of questions and I tried to give her all the right answers. We had dinner in an opulent dining room with overhanging chandeliers, and Wynn's lived up to its billing. Kathleen was fascinated with my table manners. I was very hungry and I 'cleaned my plate', as my mother would have put it. This led to some amusing comments which lightened the atmosphere and established a 'mood music' that would be continued later in the cinema. The night was a great success and indeed we had our first real kiss …

The two of us were standing face-to-face in the driveway of her home after we returned that night close to midnight, and at least one of us was trembling in anticipation. The kiss landed safely on her lips, though both sets of eyes were tightly shut and only the nearby street lamps illuminated the scene. We were mindful of the tactile sensations of closeness, of our hands brushing and the light pressure of my knee on the floating fabric of her skirt, as we sought to maintain the barrier distance for fear of failure. The solemn, unsmiling expressions on both of our faces as we drew apart again affirmed this eternal rite as serious business, to be recorded in the diary as a two-word entry with exclamation mark – 'first kiss!'. It was an important landmark in our romance, to be recalled now half a century later in print.

Despite the early progress, our courtship was slow and tentative that first year, with frequent highs and lows. Part of the reason for this was that our paths would no longer naturally cross so often in our respective routines of classes and pre-med tutorials in Botany and Zoology. I soon realised I had rivals, and at times would not get to see Kathleen for a while – only to be compelled every now and then to try to reignite the relationship by throwing pebbles late evenings at her bedroom window. Luckily this seemed to renew her ardour!

My declared interest in poetry and literature, while genuine, was also an attempt to impress Kathleen and to show her I too was into ardour. My cause was perversely advanced one day when, on an early-morning ride into class, as I was trying to catch up with her on the descent down North Avenue, I careered over the handlebars of my bike and into the garden wall of her uncle's house, sustaining a nasty head wound. Denis Donoghue, the said uncle, was then Professor of Modern English and American Literature at UCD. Kathleen knocked on the door and we were met by a tall, imposing man who recognised her. I stood gingerly beside her, holding a handkerchief to a head wound. I don't recall exactly what happened next but my vague memory was that the professor was kind and empathetic before he sent us on our way. This dramatic coincidence did not cement our relationship or further my literary pretensions, but it was a small milestone that gave me a foothold into her family. Her mother was an English teacher, which helped, and as I have said, she and I got on very well from the start. I would exploit that relationship on many future occasions during our courting years, in order to shore up my love life with Kathleen. I got to know Kathleen's sisters as well – Pat and Joan – who would also unwittingly help me through the barren times.

And there would be barren times. I was a callow, inexperienced country boy from the Bog of Allen, who was very shy to boot, and knew little about the conventions of modern dating at the time. Kathleen, on the other hand, was outgoing, fun-loving and socially very confident, and as a relatively sophisticated city girl and former pupil of Mount Anville, well-versed in the rituals and etiquette of romance. Unsurprisingly, she attracted the attentions of a number of male admirers, at least two of whom threatened to become serious prospects at one point. But luckily for me, I think Mrs McGarry, Pat and Joan were all firmly in my camp and favoured my more low-key attributes and personality as a good match for Kathleen.

2

THE ROMANCE

September 1967

Dear Finbar,

Here I am sitting in Emer's flat in Edinburgh. It's a tiny flat with two small beds. I spent last night squashed into the tiniest bed you ever saw, with P. Duffy. She wears hundreds of curlers at night and they kept sticking into me. I couldn't sleep a wink and I was thinking of you all night.

September 1967

Dear Kathleen,

I miss you and your letter had me in tears again. I hope you had a great time in Edinburgh and behaved yourself, and were not pulling up your 'tights' when everybody was looking, or swinging your legs in the air for notice.

The next few years were a rollercoaster for us both. Medical school moved from Belfield to Earlsfort Terrace in the city centre. The sedate bicycle rides were over and the pace of life changed. I bought a Honda 50 motorbike and two helmets: one for me and one for her. I hung in there with our fledging relationship, but no longer felt in charge of events – though the motorbike did give me some leverage. She was very fond of it and enjoyed sharing its passenger seat with Joan, her youngest sister, who would unwittingly assist my courtship by asking Kathleen at the end of each outing when our next date was due. Other romantic liaisons occurred for both of us around this time but hers were more significant. Adding to my disadvantage, we were geographically separated during term holidays, working in part-time jobs in Ireland and the USA to earn some money to pay our way. It was only the 'love letters' that kept us together during these coming-of-age years, and four-page epistles were the norm, though she always packed more words into hers. At the time, they were an easier and more productive means of communication, as well as much less expensive than the telephone. The mighty pen cuts to the chase once more!

Holding on to our special relationship demanded some kind of proactive initiative on my part, and this came in the guise of a soppy handwritten poem that would only get plaudits if it was composed by a five-year-old. It was the opening salvo from a dreamer with flat tyres, hoping to breathe new life into the romance. I had forgotten I wrote poems for her 50 years ago, until I very recently retrieved this literary gem from a shoebox she had hidden in one of her wardrobes. She kept them all but never told me, probably because she had forgotten them also. I cannot remember if I composed this one myself or plagiarised it from a poem I had read. It sounds very much like it was my own work!

> *To Kathleen:*
> *Her love is not a soldier,*
> *Her love is but a boy.*
> *Her dreams are not of soldiers,*
> *Her dreams – of little boys.*
> *Her wish is not for splendour,*
> *Her wish is but for joy.*
> *Of dreams and of blossoms,*
> *Of flowers and of toys.*
> *Finbarr [sic], Friday 11 p.m., 29 November 1968*

Our love letters were sent at intervals over the following years. An examination of the contents of the shoeboxes revealed there were far more of mine than hers. The temperature of the romance in retrospect could be gauged by their tone and content. Subliminal communications were lost on her and an important message could only be delivered with clarity in written form. On most occasions it had no effect on her behaviour. She ignored my frequent advice on her deportment and would continue to do so throughout the rest of her life!

Intimate letters are once-off conflated expressions of love, to be read once and never seen or spoken of again. Kathleen's letters to me during this time were equally soppy and immature, but not out of place in the culture of the sixties. Student love letters are best forgotten but did play a vital part in our formation as a couple. 'I hope you are writing lots of iambic pentameter and thinking about me and are working like mad in the cause of *hedgeumication,*' she wrote on one occasion during her lunch break in the Paperback Centre bookstore on Suffolk Street in Dublin.

30 December 1968, Edenderry
Kathleen, Happy New Year, dear. Last year was the happiest year of my life, all because I knew somebody wanted me and thought I was a nice guy to know.

9 July 1969, Teaneck, New Jersey
Dear Finbar, love, thanks for your lovely letter. I was much happier leaving when I had it to bring with me and all the lovely things you said in it to remember and make me happy. In case you can't read the ending, it says, 'All my love to Fin from Kack'.

13 October 1970, Mount Merrion
Dear Kathleen, I am listening to Bobby Goldsboro on the radio singing 'Honey', and I am dreaming of my honey in the Hodges Figgis bookshop in Galway. I miss you.

Spiky green shadows and white paint
rolling trees and no wind
as I peer through the lace window.
(from F. Lennon, 'anthology' of poems)

9 September 1971, Pensacola, Florida
Finbar, love, I am sitting alone in my room and I don't like being on my own and you so far away in St Louis. So, don't be surprised if I ring you up at all hours of the day and night if I get really too lonely altogether.

The romance survived the student years but the bigger tests were ahead of us. Kathleen graduated with honours and was marked out for a successful career in medicine. She had now more than simply 'a neat appearance, good address and a pleasant social manner', as recorded in that psychology test report back in 1966. The same test had also confirmed that she was in the top 3 per cent of her peer group in abstract reasoning and in the top 15 per cent in verbal reasoning. Well, I took some comfort in the fact she could not write poetry!

Once we graduated, the simple pleasures of student life all changed. It became a competitive world overnight. We saw less of each other and worked in different hospitals and on separate rotas. I was never going to become an Oliver St John Gogarty clone overnight, but dreaming had its moments – though I did wonder if my plan to change from traditional iambic pentameter to free verse might be a bridge too far and if Kathleen would lose interest in my musings. It did not take long to realise that my 'literary and philosophic gifts' would not be enough to hold on to her, and that my Gogarty persona, which was to surface from time to time in our future life together, would have to wait til another day! If I was going to match Kathleen's other romantic prospects, I needed to move up a gear and stop pining for my simple childhood days. Moving and shaking in the sixties and seventies, though not my forte, was an act that required a suitable vehicle, or 'fancy car', as it was called then. In my case, it had to be sufficiently flamboyant and outrageous to hide the fragile innocent behind the wheel.

As an ambitious young medical student, advancing from a Honda 50 motorbike that had served me well to a Triumph Stag sports car in one major step was my way of entering the fast lane and, at the same time, debunking hierarchy – in those days such fancy cars were the sole preserve of consultants. It was a much easier upwardly mobile step for me than advancing from an SHO (senior house officer) to a registrar's post. In those heady days in old Ireland, it opened up a field of possibilities, as they say. Kathleen was also further developing her social skills and image but was not dependent on a marquee car to make an impression. In her case, a Morris Minor with red leather seats, full of junk and clutter including chocolate bars, did just fine, since it was going to be driven by a restrained free spirit in cruise control. She did, however, miss the passenger seat of the Honda, which I had discarded with some regret as I sought to increase my profile and expand my reach.

There were other girls in my life who sat behind me on the Honda or, now, beside me in the Stag. The frisson of close physical contact and their transient dependence on me was always enough to satisfy my senses and this, combined with rambling conversations on the meaning of life, adequately addressed any remaining shortfall in my emotional life. Although the young women in question might not have admitted it at the time, they were likely equally happy with these brief innocent encounters as a precursor to more demanding liaisons to come in the future.

My challenge was to catch and keep Kathleen when the time was right. But it was a risky strategy, and whenever we went out on a date in our medical training years, she would often say, 'Make up your mind, Finbar, before it is too late!' There were many 'first kisses' and false starts during those fallow years. It was not that we had reservations about marriage – we both wanted to end up together – but our career progression was a significant competing interest for both of us and a source of subliminal conflict. Kathleen's professional destiny was secure from an early stage, whereas mine was much less certain. For that reason, I was a hesitant suitor and, eventually, the fear of losing her was what prompted me to take the plunge.

Fortunately, one evening in the Mater Hospital on the north side of the city, my guardian angel finally intervened and came to my rescue. I had just performed an appendicectomy in 20 minutes to show off my surgical skills to a few female medical students, when all of a sudden I realised that Kathleen was my number one and I began to shake, for fear I would lose her. I returned to throwing pebbles at her bedroom window with greater velocity and sense of purpose. By this time, I was no longer living with my aunt and was sharing a house elsewhere in the city with some of my fellow trainee doctors but when I did visit my aunt and would catch sight of Kathleen's car in the driveway of her parents' house nearby, I'd know that she was there that evening and would renew my efforts with the pebbles.

Eventually Kathleen responded to the persistence of my woeful wooing, in part to save the window pane but also because, as she would later tell me, she knew deep down from our early days together that we were an 'item'. However, as I would also only learn later, I had very nearly been too late, as by then she was enjoying constant romantic company and had even had offers of marriage from one or two of the young, confident academic doctors that populated St Vincent's Hospital on the south side of the city.

It took me ten years to figure out what comes after a prolonged courtship. Everybody seemed to know except me, and I nearly lost the plot. Even my father, a man of few words, felt obliged to intervene at a certain point and said to me, without mentioning the noun, that it was 'time to get on with it'. We bought the ring together in the Burlington Arcade in London's Mayfair and got engaged in early summer 1977 before anything else went off the rails. I clearly recall a sense of relief when walking hand in hand in London that summer with my 'dear ring left-fingered one', as the greeting went in a letter she received from her sister Pat following her engagement.

Most Irish weddings are made in heaven and arranged for years in advance. However, in our case, I think we were both anxious to get married quickly once I had finally popped the question: she because of her concern I might change my mind, and me because I finally realised how fortunate I was that she had said yes and that it was my last chance to 'catch her'.

We were married on 1 October 1977. Kathleen enlisted her mother to take charge of the wedding arrangements:

Dear Ma,

Thanks for the letter. The men's outfit is black tails, pinstripe trousers with waistcoats, no hats, no gloves. Finbar will do. I think we must have proper cars, especially to collect us from the chapel. If it is cheaper just to hire for collecting from the chapel, that's OK. The flower plan is OK. We must have professional photographer. I will arrange music sheet for organist. I don't want a red carpet. Please don't send invitations until Friday 2 September. I will arrange tables in hotel on Friday 30 September. Finbar to organise disco for about £35. Please arrange hair-do appointment on Saturday 1 October at 9:30 a.m. and eyelash appointment as well. Joan can do that.

Love,

Kat.

'Granny Garry' was streetwise and got most things sorted with the minimum of fuss. The marriage ceremony was in University College Church in St Stephen's Green and the wedding breakfast was in the Royal Hibernian Hotel, one of Dublin's premier hotels at the time (now long gone, its 'last farewell' menu having been served on 11 February 1982). Flowers can cause more trouble than they are worth, and Granny Garry thought most arrangements made up by florists were silly, artificial and expensive. She organised the display with the sexton who agreed that she would bring the flowers to him the day before the wedding and that he would suitably arrange them in the church on the day. She was also keen to ensure we were aware of the convention that the McGarry parents would be responsible for the costs of the breakfast and told Kathleen she would prefer if I did not contribute. We worked around that and everyone was happy, especially after my uncle, Bishop Lennon, agreed to conduct the church ceremony.

Our wedding menu – which comprised *hors d'oeuvre*, consommé soup, roast beef, apple flan, coffee and petits fours with sherry, wine and champagne – cost IR£10.60 per person. The catering manager wrote to Kathleen on 3 August to acknowledge her request to have carrots and celery served at the meal – a sign that even then she was aware that vegetables were part of a healthy diet! One hundred people attended at a cost of IR£1,060. One of the many telegrams we received on the day was from one of Kathleen's old boyfriends, who could not wait any longer for her and who was also my friend – hence his words: 'We always knew you would do it, if you lived long enough.'

We had saved IR£1,700 for the wedding. The relatives gave us another IR£300 in lieu of presents. It was enough to clear all our bills. We still came out with a positive balance, thanks to six tea/coffee sets, five sets of Waterford glasses, various items of cutlery, decanters, pottery, clocks, a coal scuttle and an electric blanket from Dennis Liston, one of Kathleen's classmates.

Everything went to plan and we lived happily ever after. Though a rocky testing ground, our unconventional, on-again/off-again, decade-long romantic apprenticeship prepared us for our future together, and in the years to come, our lengthy, unsocial working hours ensured we kept the faith and henceforth had eyes only for each other.

3

EARLY PROFESSIONAL LIFE

*Medicine has taken up a lot of my life up to now. I graduated
in UCD in 1972, where I met my husband Finbar, a classmate.
We spent our training years in Dublin, London and Edmonton,
Alberta. We got married in 1977. David, our eldest child, was
born in 1980.*

*In 1983 we settled back in Ireland, Finbar as a surgeon
in Our Lady of Lourdes Hospital in Drogheda and me, a
physician with a special interest in cardiology, in Our Lady's
Hospital, Navan. I came to Navan from Canada. I had been
offered a big job in Dublin but Finbar, who had followed me
all around the world, said the Navan job was handier for
his post in Drogheda. And so I followed him to Navan and it
has worked out well for both of us! Our home in Collon, Co.
Louth, was equidistant from both hospitals.*

*When I started to work in Navan there was no CCU, no
ICU, no ultrasound imaging, no CT scan, no ECG room
and no stress ECG service – and not enough staff. What*

kept me going over the thirty-one years were the friends and wonderful colleagues I had throughout the hospital. When I arrived there, I received a great welcome though I overheard one of my new consultant colleagues remark, 'The last thing we need is a female married cardiologist with a child.' When I went on three further statutory maternity leaves, he wondered out loud whether there was 'something in the water'!

Kathleen was a prized student in St Vincent's Hospital and won its prestigious Bellingham Gold Medal in Clinical Medicine in her final medical year. She was also a prized doctor and spent most of her early training years in St Vincent's, where she made a significant contribution to the hospital's academic and social life. I spent the same amount of training time in the Mater Hospital, but there was not much I could lay claim to, apart from a shared collegial interest in sport. Both establishments were independent Catholic voluntary hospitals and were well resourced and managed. The junior doctor rotas were demanding but the senior collegial support and supervision was good, and we learned fast. We had decided on our specialty interests at the end of the intern year. Kathleen's was general medicine/cardiology. Abstract reasoning was not my forte and so I opted for surgery.

Hard work and dedication were required to make the grade in both specialties and there were exams along the way that had to be passed to progress to the next level. Kathleen had no problems but I had some failed attempts that blotted my copybook, and I had difficulty keeping up with her as we moved from SHO to registrar jobs. She was writing papers for medical journals, while I was spending most of my time performing appendicectomies – and after removing a certain number, there were no extra academic points to be gained in removing any more. When I was scouting around London for a less sought-after registrar's job in the East End, I used to occasionally try to impress the interview board during the getting-to-know-you preamble by mentioning my wife's recent appointments to Great Ormond Street and Hammersmith hospitals. It did not work, so I gave up this ploy and was eventually appointed to Queen Mary's Hospital in Stratford.

Kathleen's prospects of becoming a consultant soared after her appointments to two prestigious London hospitals. Meanwhile, I was on a 1-in-2 rota (on call after-hours every other day) in a very busy, poorly resourced hospital that was on emergency call. I was now removing kidneys and stomachs but not making much academic progress, as again these organ removals unfortunately did not enhance my CV. I often fell asleep on the Underground on my way back to the flat and missed my stop, and so any opportunity for extracurricular study or writing papers was lost. Two of my consultant mentors in the Mater kept in touch with me and promised to support me when the national senior registrar posts were advertised. I was happy to bask in Kathleen's success and, despite both our very demanding jobs, we enjoyed our two years in London.

We returned to Dublin in July 1979. She was appointed a research fellow in pharmacology at the Royal College of Surgeons, and, in an unusual year when six posts were vacant, I was lucky to be appointed a senior registrar in surgery on a rotation that commenced in St Vincent's and continued in the Mater. In November 1980, we were delighted to welcome our first son, David, into the world.

When in early 1981 Kathleen told me she had been offered a senior resident post in clinical cardiology in Edmonton for 15 months from that July, I had to use the surgical grapevine again to secure my first academic appointment in the University of Alberta. David of course came to Canada with us. Our training years ended following those two assignments. She could have got a consultant post anywhere, and indeed did, but after she married me, she realised her options were more limited if we wanted to be together full-time. She now had to lower her sights and follow me for the first time in her professional life!

After flying home from Edmonton for two unsuccessful consultant interviews, I finally struck it lucky in Drogheda. I was offered the post of consultant general surgeon in a late-evening telephone call with the hospital administrator, a nun – on the proviso that I gave her a verbal undertaking there and then that I would live within three miles of the hospital. The only sensible answer at the time was 'yes'! We had now both climbed the mountain, taken a deep breath and could look forward to the next stage of our lives with hope and trepidation.

In 1982 Kathleen had been a senior resident in University Hospital, Edmonton, in a cardiology division with five consultants and state-of-the-art medical and cardiac diagnostic equipment, including CT and ultrasound scans. Within a short space of time she had moved back home to become a single-handed general physician with a sub-specialty interest in cardiology in Our Lady's Hospital, Navan, with only basic equipment in the form of plain X-rays and ECG machines. There she was expected to be on duty 24/7 for the duration, with three trainee doctors and one experienced registrar to assist in looking after all the medical needs of a 200-bed acute general hospital. Single-handed physicians were commonplace in some of the small Irish county hospitals at the time. These were good jobs, but not attractive ones. For highly trained Irish medical specialists, the move from major university hospitals in North America to working in professional isolation in poorly resourced hospitals at home was a daunting proposition.

Our Lady's Hospital, Navan, had begun its days in 1841 as part of a workhouse set up to look after the poor and destitute of the town. The hospital had access to a doctor but was chiefly staffed by inmates of the workhouse. In 1891 the Sisters of Mercy were handed control of the hospital and a small chapel was built on the premises, which is still in use today. In 1924 the workhouse became the county hospital and the first 'consultant', a surgeon—

physician, was appointed. In 1951 the hospital was dedicated to Our Lady, Mother of God, and was officially named after her. Surgery was the first medical specialty to receive recognition in Ireland, and official consultant appointments date from 1957.

When she first arrived back in Ireland in 1983, Kathleen could have been forgiven for wondering what was so special about surgeons. They had a more prominent presence in the smaller Irish hospitals in the 1970s and 80s, not only because there were more of them in such hospitals but also because most had mercurial and robust personalities. Hence surgeons tended to have a self-designated say in how the hospital was managed and, generally speaking, their directive style was helpful and welcomed. Many such smaller hospitals were managed by matrons who were also nuns, and who as such were accustomed to deferring to figures of authority.

Female consultants were uncommon in those days, and Kathleen had to adapt her 'human factor skills' to impress her surgical colleagues. At the time she was appointed in Navan, the consultant staffing complement was five surgeons (two general and three orthopaedic), two anaesthetists, one radiologist, one pathologist – and now she was joining them as the solitary consultant physician. The official bed complement was 197, though in many hospitals the numbers didn't always add up. The majority comprised orthopaedic and general surgical beds, and there were 56 general medical beds, most of which were used for acute admissions.

We had decided to rent separate houses in Navan and Drogheda for the first year because of my promise to the Medical Missionaries of Mary (MMM) who owned the hospital in Drogheda that I would reside within a three-mile radius, as I would be on a 1-in-2 rota. Since Kathleen would be on call all the time in Navan (which was about 14 miles from Drogheda), and had no idea how that was going to work out, we had no other option. It soon became clear, however, that these living arrangements were not a viable proposition for work or family life, even in the short term. I was coming over to Navan on my off-call nights to sleep, mind the baby and cuddle the physician – but that was never going to be enough to keep the show on the road!

We got some home help in Navan and started looking at houses for sale in the area. We were lucky and found one in Collon that we liked and were keen to buy. Collon was equidistant from our two places of work, and so was a good choice from that perspective too.

'Do you think you will get away with this plan, Finbar?' Kathleen asked me. The next day I was due to meet the Mother General of the MMM for afternoon tea in their administrative centre in nearby Mell. This was a privilege afforded at the time to all new consultants during their first year in post (which was effectively also a probation year).

'I have it all worked out, Kathleen. A combination of charm, praise and deference generally works on religious superiors, and

I can also use the "bishop card"!' (My uncle was then a bishop of the Kildare and Leighlin diocese).

'Don't get too smart,' she replied.

I was accompanied to the meeting by the Sister Administrator of the hospital who had offered me the job in the first place. She sat some distance away from the Mother General and me as we conversed.

'Have you found a place to live?' the senior nun asked, after exchanging the usual pleasantries.

'Well, Mother General, you won't believe it, but we have just put down a deposit on a lovely house in Collon, within 100 yards of the MMM's original mother house and novitiate in the village there.'

'That's wonderful,' she replied, as she turned to beam approvingly at her colleague in the corner. And the rest is history.

In 1983 we purchased Greenlawns, a period terraced house on the main street in Collon, a village on a busy commuter route along the Dublin–Derry road. The house is the very opposite of an imposing residence and has often been described as a ramshackle, 'all over the place' house with old-world, idiosyncratic features inside and outside. There was no front door in the conventional sense, but a gate door leading to a side entrance to the house. Inside there was a pavilion-style living room, a sun lounge and five bathrooms of various shapes and sizes, one of which we only discovered some days after taking up residence. The old Georgian windows at the front permitted fresh air to circulate all year round, even when shut and bolted. The constant passing traffic was always clearly audible. Outside there was a cattle grid at the front entrance and pleasure gardens at the rear, with high hedges and tall trees providing seclusion, and multiple fruit trees. There was plenty of play and living space inside and outside, and we thought it would be a good family house.

Collon is a small, sleepy village with an interesting history, in spite of not being on the tourist map. It has two churches and a Cistercian monastery and was the home of John Foster, the last Speaker of the Irish House of Commons at the end of the eighteenth century. After the Second World War, the village was a haven for Russian émigrés, and even the odd spy if one is to believe local folklore. One of the former, Nikolai Couriss, who had close links with the imperial family, established a Russian-language school in the old courthouse in the village square in 1946. It was rumoured that the three famous British spies Philby, Burgess and McClean came to Collon to learn the language and spent time in the school. This story is explored in the book *Blood Relative* by Michael Gray (published in 1998 by Weidenfeld and Nicolson), who established that a Count Tolstoy and Couriss were friends from their student days and subsequently lived close together for a number of years in the village.

Our house deeds confirmed that Greenlawns was the

dwelling of Count Mikhail Pavlovich Kutuzov-Tolstoy and his wife from 1951 until 1957. The count was a remote descendant of Tsar Nicholas I. The house was also home to some Tolstoy family heirlooms, as has been reported in the press, including three leather-bound volumes of *War and Peace*. Our current housekeeper, Rosemary, was employed by the countess as a home help when she was 14 years old, and recalls her love of cooking and gardening, as well as her charitable work in the village and surrounding area. In his autobiography, *The Story of my Life*, published in 1986, Mikhail Pavlovich Kutuzov-Tolstoy recounts how he and his wife were expelled from Hungary in 1951 and left Budapest on a truncated Orient Express comprising an engine, a restaurant car and one completely empty sleeping car. They obtained resident permits in Ireland and bought Greenlawns in Collon, 'a pleasant old house, ivory covered, with a big courtyard behind it, and a walled garden of about an acre'. They spent 'six uneventful years' in Collon. Myriam, the countess, apparently never liked the village: 'It had no possibilities, no attractions for our guests …' She must have been glad when an inheritance from her mother allowed them to eventually move to a bigger house in Delgany, County Wicklow.

Although we employed four successive live-in nannies/ housekeepers during the years our children were growing up, our two honorary childminders from the very beginning were close neighbours we met on the day we arrived in Collon in 1983. Paddy and May Ward were respected elders in the community at the time. He had already retired from active duty as a skilled tradesman before we had commenced our terms of service, but he was still alert in mind and body. For the first time in our married life we were known locally as 'Doctor and Missus Lennon', but the use of these titles was confined to the village and they had no recognition or currency beyond.

Paddy passed his competency tests with 'the Missus' without formal interview and was retained on a long-term contract as houseman and head of operations on the 'Greenlawns estate'. She and he agreed terms and conditions without any reference to 'Himself'. Paddy was the proverbial jack-of-all-trades, and there was no task too difficult or complex for him to manage. Apart from the childminding duties he shared with May, he looked after all our electric, plumbing, carpentry and gardening needs. He and Kathleen were very fond of each other. He arrived each weekday morning to guide her out of the driveway onto the main road and would stop the traffic until she was safely on her way to Navan. He then spent most of the morning doing odd jobs in the house and garden. He walked the children to primary school and home again, but, on the latter journey, not before calling into May for lemonade and buns. He was the second man in Kathleen's married life and lived to 103. May lived to be 100 years old.

We moved in around mid-summer after employing a young live-in nanny/housekeeper to mind David. We bought some of the furniture that came with the house and quickly set about getting three or four rooms in order. At the time, Greenlawns had an unreliable telephone system and the handset in our bedroom had an extra-long flex connected to a wall socket, demanding care and attention at night to ensure it did not become disconnected during toilet visits. Unfortunately, I tripped over it one night within a few weeks of taking up residence and could have foreshortened my career by 30 years if not for God's grace and my professional fleet-footedness and subsequent manual dexterity.

That evening's events also included a truly surreal moment and a night in the theatre. I was on call and a young man had been admitted to the hospital with a serious abdominal stab injury. During the night Kathleen woke me – I had just fallen back to sleep after my tussle with the telephone cord.

'Finbar, somebody is throwing stones at the window, and it is not you!'

It was the parish priest, and when I opened the window, he shouted that there was an emergency in the hospital and they had been unable to contact me by phone. I drove the seven-mile journey in the time it would normally have taken a nun to drive three. I arrived to the sight of the big hands of an orthopaedic surgeon compressing multiple large pads to staunch the bleeding in the patient's open abdomen. Two hours later we had it under control, and the patient survived. The following day the Sister Administrator met me in the corridor and inquired how I was settling into our house in Collon …

4

ON THE FRONT LINE

The same kinds of emergency medical cases present to and are admitted to the hospital in Navan as to the major teaching hospitals in Dublin. Patients and their relatives expect and deserve the same standard of care and the same outcomes in both locations. I spent a huge amount of time throughout my 31 years in post trying to improve resources and increase the staffing levels of senior and junior doctors in the medical unit. I was constantly writing letters to hospital managers and senior executives in the Regional Health Authority, in addition to making representations and lobbying local politicians and government ministers. With the support of my professional college, things gradually improved but it took ages. I was a single-handed physician for 13 years. Now there are five on-call physicians. There still remain great disparities in hospital services across the country.

Plans to close or downgrade community hospitals like Navan and centralise acute and complex care in a number of large hospitals have been a source of great concern to the local community for decades. The current plan to reorganise services into a number of large hospital groups, which makes sense, is stifled by local politics and is not yet fully in place. I think it will be best for Navan in the long-term as long as they retain and develop what works well here.

Important meetings are feature events in all small hospitals in Ireland. There are, in fact, no other types of meetings. Kathleen attended her first administrative consultant committee meeting in Navan hospital in early 1983. The minutes record that she was formally welcomed by the chairperson and later note that a project team for the development of a new hospital had just been set up. Her only contribution at the meeting was to state that 'a room was needed for ECG examinations'.

The minutes of that meeting also reveal that the total budget allocation for Our Lady's Hospital in Navan in 1983 was IR£4.8 million and, as was normal practice at the time, the breakdown of its allocation was notified in advance to the consultants. Of this, IR£2.9 million was for staff salaries. Included in the remainder was IR£43,000 for turf, IR£68,000 for meat, IR£15,000 for milk, IR£12,600 for potatoes and vegetables, IR£800 for oratory supplies and IR£300 for entertainment. The state's priorities in straitened times were pay, food and drink (milk) and heat, which could not be faulted. Also provided for was some token nourishment for the soul through the religious and entertainment allocations!

Some weeks later, Kathleen and I discussed her own professional predicament, and she showed me some of the correspondence from the meeting. We agreed the hospital budget was insufficient and was the limiting factor on additional staff recruitment. I felt, as she did, that that year's proposed plan for the hospital was not realistic. She was anxious to do something constructive to highlight her vulnerability as a single-handed medical consultant but did not want to upset her health-board employer.

'If you write to management, keep a record of the correspondence.'

'OK, Finbar, but will it make any difference?'

'Yes, Kathleen, it will. Some time down the road they will come back to you for advice and direction.'

The tone of one of the first letters she sent to the senior executive responsible for the region's hospital services is reflected in this extract: *'I am a little worried that in the current economic climate, the proposed second medical consultant post will be frozen. The board already pay locum services for my time off and I feel it would be better if the money went towards funding the second consultant post.'*

Both of us spent our working lives dealing with science

and humanity and applying the related facts and foibles to our care management plan. In small hospitals at the time, patients were fortunate to receive a consultant-provided and -delivered service. In Navan, Kathleen was alone on the front line and directed the care plan from admission to discharge. There were no hierarchical layers of doctors then between the consultant and the patient. This ensured a more meaningful doctor–patient interaction, and a closer empathetic bond was established that served both parties well. Unfortunately, this was only sustainable on a short-term basis, as the workload was far too onerous for a single-handed physician.

Kathleen and I never worked together in the same hospital and lived totally separate professional lives. I knew none of her patients, she none of mine. The only cross-discipline interaction that occurred between us was in bed at night, whenever we got phone calls from our respective hospitals. She would always pick up the phone first.

'It's a bleeder – that's for you,' she would say with relief.

There were times when I was abrupt and rude, as I gave curt management instructions to the unfortunate junior doctor on the other end of the line. After these calls, she would berate me for my manners, then there would be a silent pause before she added her frequent follow-up rejoinder: 'I think you should go in and see that patient.'

By contrast, there were often occasions when, after a lengthy bedtime review of a case with her on-call junior doctor and her subsequent management advice, delivered in a gentle, collegial manner, she was still concerned about the patient as she put the phone down.

I would nudge her and invariably reassure her: 'You don't need to go in.'

She regarded such interventions as my being smart and unhelpful. And she usually did go in because she knew that the pressure and responsibility on the single on-call junior doctor was too much. Nevertheless, we were both hard taskmasters, albeit one of us gentle, considerate and firm, and the other incisive, testy and sometimes unreasonable. Like most physicians, Kathleen was what is referred to as a 'cognitive' doctor, best described as a critical thinker who has to establish the diagnosis and develop an overall care plan by forensic assessment of all the relevant data. Hence, she always had a little more time to ponder before making decisions. By contrast, the surgeon's main focus and interest is the procedure or operation. I actually believed I was also a cognitive doctor, although thinking and pondering is not a forte of many busy surgeons, whose default position is the operating theatre, where all will be revealed.

When Kathleen was on call, it often meant a night without sleep. It was a 30-minute journey to Navan on poor roads. On those occasions, it was also a night without sleep for me, as I was left to mind the baby. There were many times when we both had to go in – she to put in a pacemaker, or me to perform an emergency operation – particularly in the early days, when the junior staff had little experience and there were so few of them. If we were both called out at the same time, the live-in nanny was there to take over with David. We had a fax machine in the study downstairs, whose main purpose was to receive ECG recordings from Navan to determine whether the acute medical presentations had arrhythmias or had had heart attacks. I was dispatched from the bed to fetch these readings but this 'advanced transmission technology', while helpful in some cases, did not prevent many late-night and early-morning commutes by Kathleen to the hospital. Aside from the late-night hospital phone calls and the basic exchanges we had about them, our bedtime conversations were always short. She learned very little from me about surgery and I was too tired to listen to her long medical cases. Once 'lactic acidosis' was mentioned, I was off!

The doctor knows best if he or she delivers the service first-hand. And that's what we had to do during the first half of our consultant lives. We made mistakes but we were at the coalface 24/7, and our name was above the bed. At that time, we did morning ward rounds every day. Most of the clinical problems were picked up in a timely way and then we had to fix them. There was no one else to call on. The sooner the problem was discovered and fixed, the better the outcome for the patient, and that truism is just as valid today.

Taking a history and doing a physical examination were the primary sources of information about a patient's condition at the time. Basic, plain X-rays were available but only a limited number of blood tests were performed out of hours. The dependence in modern-day practice on investigations to provide the diagnosis and determine the follow-up treatment has downgraded the patient history and physical examination from their intended preeminent role. Many patients are put at risk of over-investigation and over-treatment as a result. In truth, tests, investigations and X-rays are complementary aids to diagnosis and each provides a distinct and important contribution to the care management plan. We relied greatly on patient histories and physical examinations for a large number of our years in practice, and the weight given to each depended very much on the individual clinician. Kathleen would often remark to me that she was surprised how little attention would be given to physical examination in follow-up clinical reviews. And in this, she was, of course, comparing her own approach to that of her peers. On the other hand, my own experience was that surgeons paid much more attention to the physical examination and much less to the gathering of the patient history, as they believed action – their own – spoke louder than words.

The mission statements of all developed health services today include some variation on the phrase 'It's all about the patient'. Patient-centred services are based on shared decision-making between patients and their doctors. When the patient is centre stage, the dynamic, of course, changes and the doctor becomes more defensive in his or her approach. Kathleen and

I, however, worked at a time when the doctor was in charge and, accordingly, more reliance was placed on the clinical knowledge, experience and wisdom of the doctor and less on blood tests and investigations. The health algorithm carousel has flipped since then to the extent that one could be forgiven for wondering if, instead of the patients, the investigations are now centre stage.

Kathleen did both her public and private practice in Navan. There was no distinction in how the patients were treated and often no difference in their accommodation, which was in large multi-bedded 'Nightingale' wards with little or no privacy. Most of the medical inpatients were acute or emergency admissions. The physical infrastructure, facilities, basic medical equipment and medical staffing levels of the hospital were poor. On the other hand, the working environment was pleasant and the can-do attitude of staff and managers was refreshing and motivating, with everybody doing their best to deliver a good and caring service.

Not all peripheral or rural hospitals in Ireland in the 1980s were the same. Some were better than others in many respects. That is still the case today, but they are no longer stand-alone institutions and the smaller hospitals are now partnered with major teaching hospitals. The standard of care is now more uniform across the country, though significant disparities still remain. Our Lady's Hospital, Navan was, and is, a small hospital with an emergency department that continues to provide 24/7 acute medical care. It has become an outlier, as most of its peer hospitals do not provide emergency services. It has successfully resisted change and reform as a result of strong political lobbying and community support. However, this public pressure to retain acute medical services only succeeded because its accomplished medical teams consistently dispensed the correct medications and treatments to the acute general medical, cardiovascular and respiratory cases that came through its doors.

During Kathleen's tenure in Navan, knowing the private telephone numbers of the medical-consultant 'heavyweights' in Dublin was very important, as they were more than happy to provide a helping hand to their lone colleagues from outside the Pale. This medical grapevine facilitated the transfer of 'Honour's cases' (that is, difficult or complex cases) to the major centres. Kathleen was also lucky in having surgical and radiological colleagues in Navan who frequently offered unsolicited advice on how to treat difficult medical cases. Another source of advice in the smaller hospitals was the patients' relatives, who believed they should be consulted on treatment options and were at times emboldened to challenge the single-handed consultant about the management plan, which she or he had to be prepared to explain and justify on each ward round. Relatives were always present or nearby, monitoring the doctors on behalf of their family member — unlike in the bigger hospitals, where they would be asked to leave the bedside during ward rounds. Relatives and friends of the patient would keep the consultant 'honest', and on occasion the lone consultant was served well by their interest and presence.

Diseases of the heart and lungs accounted for a large proportion of the acute medical admissions to Navan, but any kind of acute medical, surgical or paediatric emergency could present to its accident and emergency department, and this happened on many occasions. Kathleen was very dependent on the junior doctors, and the smart, ambitious young trainees realised that they could get more hands-on experience by coming to Navan as part of their rotation. She quickly gained a very good reputation for teaching and supervising her trainees. The problem was that the junior staff complement was completely inadequate, and those that came got great experience, but at the cost of a very demanding and exhausting workload. They spent six months there, where they saw and did everything. They were fast learners and were good for Kathleen and eased her burden.

For her part, she knew that without them she could not maintain a safe service, and hence she began making representations to the hospital managers for more resources and more doctors. Her colleagues on the medical board supported her but the representations, while sympathetically acknowledged, did not have the desired effect. The national health budget was always stretched and, of course, the same shortcomings in staff and infrastructure were affecting similar hospitals scattered around the country. Kathleen was blessed to have a trusted and loyal lieutenant, Dr Sothy, who was a long-term registrar with a strong vocational commitment to the hospital. He shared the workload with her and, though all patients were admitted under her care until 1997, he ensured she had some downtime and family life.

The life of a junior doctor in the 70s and 80s was extremely stressful, with no such thing as days off after full nights 'on the trot'. I recall working in London every second night as a paediatric cardiac registrar on-call, and getting off at 7.00 p.m. on my night off! Stress of course gives rise to greater alcohol intake, and I often rewarded myself with a nice glass of wine or two after a long busy day.

The life of a physician who was single-handed for many years in a rural hospital in Ireland over the last 30 years was not without its stresses either. It is worth describing some of these. I had a very heavy workload, both in the hospital and at home. Everyone is subject to various scares and worries in family life, of which the illnesses of children and parents are surely the worst. Do all these factors lead to more unhealthy lifestyles, such as, for example, with less exercise and more alcohol intake?

Work–life balance was not a term used in medical – or many other – circles when we qualified in 1972. For new doctors, it was all work and very little life. Family time was in short supply, but initially, since we were single, it did not matter so much. When we both commenced our consultant practice in 1983, a 100-hour working week was commonplace. Sleep time was frequently disrupted by work and children. As a result, for many years when the children were growing up our lives were full of stress and hurry. Our routine working days often stretched into evenings, and we spent long hours on night-time call-outs – until I realised that most emergency surgical operations can safely wait until next morning and that physicians can give expert directive advice to their junior colleagues from the comfort of their beds. Notwithstanding my brainwave, we were still in effect on 24/7 call for the first 15 years. Time off and leisure activities were moving targets and happened more by chance than design. While there is no direct link between stress and cancer, there is emerging evidence that disruption to a person's circadian rhythm may increase the risk of cancer and cardiovascular diseases. Work-related stress can also lead to increased alcohol intake, and Kathleen's post-shift tipples of wine, though always moderate, may not have been prudent in the long term.

5

CALLING IT AS SHE SAW IT

When I look back now on our professional working life in both hospitals, it all appears quite shocking. Finbar was one of two general surgeons in a 340-bed hospital, dealing with emergency trauma, general and paediatric surgery. He worked on the infamous 1-in-2 on-call rota when his night duty was often very busy. It was a time when, in the absence of the facilities for tests and investigations, clinical decisions based on physical examinations and patient histories determined the management plan in many cases.

Meanwhile I was the only consultant physician in Navan, a 200-bed hospital which included a large orthopaedic unit. Theoretically I was on call all the time, and if it were not for my good fortune of meeting and working alongside Dr Sothy, a very accomplished doctor who was a long-term medical registrar in the hospital, I would not have stuck it.

The advice Irish doctors receive on taking up consultant posts in Ireland is to grin and bear with all the shortcomings in infrastructure and personnel for the first few years, and do the best you can to provide a safe and quality service. Though Kathleen was very patient and made frequent informal representations, they were to no avail and she concluded that the wait-and-see option was not a runner in Navan. Her own workload on the frontline increased year on year and she could see the demands and pressures on the junior medical staff, trying to deliver a safe, caring service to patients in a poorly resourced hospital. She began to make waves with hospital management. In spite of what television medical dramas may portray, they are often on your side. Many see the deficits and faults in the system just as you do, but they are too low in the managerial hierarchy to fix the problems. In a small hospital, it's a tight-knit medical and administrative community, and rocking the boat has to be gentle at first, even though that approach does not generally work in the short term. Shaking, screaming and shouting comes next, and that never works. The only recourse is to go back to gently rocking the boat, but with greater persistence and tenacity than before, along with an acceptance that you are in it for the long haul, often over a lifetime in practice. You can only hope that the legacy and memory you leave behind makes the difference. From very early on in her time at Navan, this was Kathleen's objective – as her correspondence confirms.

1991

We urgently need a second consultant physician and extra junior doctors to practise safely ... I realise the board is in financial difficulty but given our increased level of activity we must fund extra posts ... I enclose a letter sent to me by the junior doctors who are very critical of the poor staffing levels in the hospital ... It is not acceptable to have a single-handed consultant physician responsible for the care of 2000 emergency admissions each year.

1993

Last night at midnight there were six emergencies. Three acute admissions – a young girl with a severe diabetic coma, a lady with a heart attack and another with respiratory failure and a pneumothorax. At the same time three inpatients required urgent treatment: one with acute confusion, a second with respiratory failure and a third with ventricular tachycardia. There was only one house doctor on duty, and I had to come in and assist her and admit the patients.

... I would like to congratulate you on your appointment as Programme Manager for hospitals. Thank you for the sympathetic hearing and allocating an extra junior doctor to the medical unit.

1995
A very great problem is that we can only roster one doctor out-of-hours. Nursing staff shortages at night continue. … I need a 1:2 rota now and a 1:3 rota in time. I need to be allowed to develop my interest and expertise in cardiology.

1997
Please find enclosed all my correspondence about the unsafe situation in hospital when only one doctor can be rostered at night.

1998
I have been working here since 1983. Patients were admitted under my name every day, until Dr Sothy was employed as a locum consultant in 1997.

2002
It is very difficult to manage critically ill patients without CT facilities on site. We are still awaiting the appointment of a third consultant physician with a special interest in rheumatology.

2006
There is an urgent need to set up a medical assessment unit [MAU], as recommended by the Medical Council and the College of Physicians, and to address the inadequate numbers of medical consultants and trainee doctors.

2011

*I am writing yet again. The MAU was opened in December
2008 with a promise of two additional consultant
physicians. No progress has been made in securing these
permanent appointments.*

*… I am writing about junior doctor shortages. As you
know the number of juniors, in particular SHOs, is
inadequate with no possibility of cross-cover, given that we
are providing a 24-hour acute unselected on-call service.*

A safe service is one where patient care is not compromised by
deficits in essential resources. If patients die in hospital, as many
with acute medical conditions surely do, it should always be as a
result of their disease. Kathleen recognised the deficits in Navan
when she arrived and felt it was her professional responsibility
to seek to correct them. One of her most important ongoing
priorities was to highlight the staffing problems in the medical
unit. A fine line has to be negotiated in pursuing such an
agenda, and Kathleen's efforts were always pursued on the basis
that everybody – doctors, nurses and managers – was on the
same side. That team ethos was her great gift, and sometimes
her Achilles heel. As I had advised her very early on, she kept
copies of all her correspondence with management throughout
her 31 years' tenure. She was a hoarder by nature, but in this
case, she wanted to ensure there was a record of her efforts to

improve patient care and the working conditions of trainee doctors, that there was evidence that her persistent advocacy over the years was borne out in the changes that were made. The constant battle was a great strain on her, particularly as the case she was making on behalf of the staff and patients was strong and clearly justified. She was always seeking consensus but she also felt strongly that she had a professional duty to make her concerns known.

The Irish health service has been in difficulty for half a century. The expectations citizens have of it are understandable and valid. The current performance benchmarks for measuring primary (GP) and secondary (hospital) care services are realistic. Healthcare staff cannot perform and meet their responsibilities unless the service is adequately funded, resourced and managed and their own vital contribution is acknowledged and valued. Structural reform is the only recourse available to management to respond to the relentless, ever-spiralling costs of healthcare provision.

The clinical and management staff working on the front line need to understand that the system will not fix itself. Constant efforts to advocate for and encourage local change will result in incremental progress but the job will never end. Those in charge have to be able to identify the people in the workforce who can help: those who can provide wise and prudent advice and have no personal agenda, 'no axe to grind and no chip on the shoulder'. They need to seek out individuals who have knowledge and experience, who are working daily at the coalface and who know what is wrong and how to fix it. They require good listeners who understand the constraints of managers, the vagaries of colleagues and the parlous financial situation that is the constant bedfellow of the healthcare system. They must seek out those who are willing to fight the ongoing battles with gusto and to lose with grace, knowing that if the cause is worth the candle, their opportunity to highlight it will come again. When all is going awry, they are the ones who will stand up and support the staff, laugh at the nonsense and make another cup of tea. Kathleen was such a person.

6

'WHAT DO YOU THINK OF MY LEGS?'

Amazingly in our busy working lives, we were fortunate to have three more children. After David came Ruth, Peter and Stephen, and this was a source of joy and contentment: a busy family life and all that goes with rearing children, including the Wednesday afternoon rugby and netball games. Surprisingly none of the four children showed any interest in a medical career, I suppose not fancying the busy working commitments and disruptive lifestyles of their parents. We were fortunate to have the support of my wonderful parents. Kevin was an engineer and the son of two school teachers in Drumraney in Co. Westmeath and my mother was an English teacher originally from Warrenpoint in Co. Down.

For me, Kathleen's remarkable abilities and gifts as a parent and mother transcended even her not inconsiderable achievements as a medic. The wonder was she was always conscious of the mismatch. She was fully aware of the conflicting demands of these very challenging roles, yet could live comfortably in both worlds; she was somehow able to give of herself generously and without reserve, both to our children and to her patients.

The responsibility of parents has always been the same: to protect and be there for their children. It is both an active and passive role, where in the latter sense you lead by example, hoping they will see and understand the values you try to live by. Kathleen had the insight to see that goodness in her parents and was always kind, generous and grateful for the opportunities and encouragement they gave her. She knew she had done them proud, and her achievements in medicine were a source of joy and contentment to them. They were always there when she needed them, not beside her, but calmly and quietly observing from a distance, ready to assist and advise, able to cheer and console. Their parental generosity was bestowed in equal measure to each of her sibs. That was the same benchmark she applied in her lifetime to all four of our children. She believed those halcyon family days of hers could be recreated by us for our own children, to be cherished in turn by them and the next generation when the time came.

The team ethos that Kathleen displayed and practised in her working life and, later, as the head of our household and heart of our family life came from her own upbringing. Her family was a close-knit unit, where each of the seven members, parents and children, was comfortable in each other's company as they acted out their roles within its hierarchy. The seven Lennons of my own family were not so demonstrably close but we were always there for each other, no less a family unit – more distant and self-reliant, perhaps, yet fully aware of the important bonds of kinship. We Lennon sibs were all alike in that sense, so it must be something in our genetic make-up that is responsible for my characteristic tincture of stoicism and social aloofness. It is often remarked by those that knew him that I am very like my late father, and it is a wonderful compliment that I cherish. Nevertheless, I am grateful that it was Kathleen's good genes that shaped our own children in some important respects. They certainly did not learn their social skills from Dad!

Kathleen was a good friend to have at one's side and she enjoyed company. She was unpretentious and had an easy, natural way about her. Many of her friends, both male and female, were lifelong and she was devoted to them. She met them as often as her work, family and social calendar permitted, but was equally happy using old and new means of communication to keep in touch. She was very fond of handwritten letters and cards and would use all the available writing space to pack in every item of news and gossip before signing off with smiley faces and 'x's. While she used 'the mobile' for business, the landline phone in Collon was her gateway to the world, and she used it to excess, especially once she began winding down her work commitments.

Whenever one of Kathleen's special friends phoned, she would ensure that I was out of earshot, and if I was nearby, she would wave me away with a firm hand gesture and a frown. Later, during her illness, I would come to welcome their calls with open arms. She liked to talk and so did most of them! I was always happy to leave her to it and disappear to the garden to continue my hermetic existence. One of these long-standing and loquacious friends was an old surgical boyfriend from St Vincent's Hospital, who was the only other man in her life who could send her into fits of laughter. I always knew when he was on the phone, even from the garden. I was never concerned because she was a good Catholic wife, but more than that, I knew she loved me and was very happy with me and so would never leave me. He never left her either! However, I did get upset on occasions when I returned 30 or 40 minutes later to see her with her ear still glued to the handset. She would purposely avoid eye contact because she knew my face would be contorted in exasperation and my hands waving wildly out of sync. She would try to get even by seeking any rare opportunity to catch me engaged in a call myself, listening to one of my three long-winded friends. Her way of handling this was entirely different to mine. She would pull a seat over or lie on the bed beside me and smile, laugh and tickle me to distract me from the conversation. And since I was generally in listening mode only, I would sometimes pass over the handset to her and simply leave the room!

An equal source of enjoyment for Kathleen was a shopping

expedition. She loved a bargain. In 1950s Ireland, anything for 19s. 99d. was a bargain, but in the new millennium no Irish woman worth her salt would be fooled by that old marketing ploy. Any markdown, particularly on clothes, caught her eye and she would buy the item regardless of colour, fit or need. Any outfit on sale for half price sent her into ecstatic overdrive, and multiples would be bought in one go. They were stashed in the car boot, driven home at giddy speed, unloaded surreptitiously when I was out of sight and purposefully stored in faraway wardrobes throughout the house, never to surface again. Over the years some of them were distributed as gifts to family and friends on special occasions. Since Kathleen's death, literally hundreds of 'bargains' have been retrieved by her sisters, Joan and Pat, and our daughter, Ruth, many of them still pristine in their packaging, having never been worn.

In the very early days, before I realised how fashion-conscious she was, I bought the occasional dress for her in a local drapery shop. During the most recent wardrobe clear-out, I found one such dress with the price tag still hanging from one of its lapels. It must have been an expensive dress for me to have left it attached. Kathleen's interest in the world of fashion commenced soon after her appointment to Navan hospital, after she visited the leading regional fashion store in Athboy in County Meath. She quickly identified the second-tier fashion houses across the country, many of which stocked clothes from leading designers at discounted prices. The possibility of a bargain always added an extra frisson for her. She struck gold when she found the John Bentley line in the Athboy store. So you can only imagine her delight when she discovered that the founders and designers of the clothes that appealed so much to her were none other than our wonderful neighbours in Collon, John and Michael, who lived not 50 yards from Greenlawns.

John and Michael had set up their rag-trade business in the early 1990s in Collon House, which dated from 1740 and was the former home of Anthony Foster, Lord Chief Baron of the Exchequer, and father of John Foster, the last Speaker of the Irish House of Commons. John our neighbour was a disciple of Giorgio Armani and soon became Kathleen's personal dresser. She 'modelled' his summer and winter collections at her social outings, and her rewards included bargain deals on his first clothes off the catwalk each season. Another of John and Michael's claims to fame are the garden and dinner parties they host for their 'very best friends' in the beautiful setting of Collon House, which they have restored to its former glory – and Kathleen was always top of their list of invitees. In return for regular invitations and the best seats in the house, we were both happy to give freely of our professional services and provided periodic advice on the respective states of John's and Michael's health. The arrangement worked wonders for all four of us!

It never took Kathleen long to get ready for any professional or social event – as long as I remembered to switch on the hot water in good time. Her preparation commenced with a wash. She preferred a hot bath to a shower, and indeed her nightly bath was a routine she rarely missed. She often spent less than a minute in it completing all her ablutions, despite its preparation taking over an hour. First the two heat switches on the old immersion heater were turned on, generally by me, and then, before bedtime, she'd fill the tub to the brim. After alighting from the bath, she would quickly pull the plug and all 80 gallons of water were subsequently dispatched down the drain with a loud gurgling fanfare of sound. She was never into cosmetics, apart from Chanel No. 5 perfume, which she'd squirt liberally on head and shoulders, arms and legs. I bought her small bottles as presents, which were always well received. Part of the reason for small bottles was to try to reduce her consumption! A much less costly skin cosmetic that was the rage in her Mount Anville schooldays was just as effective but had lost its allure in the modern market and was no longer on sale. Going by the name Heavenly Lotion, it was described in a Dublin social magazine in 1966 as 'a miracle worker for rejuvenating dry skin' and was advertised alongside a photograph of that season's debutantes, including Kathleen at her school coming-out ball.

Most of her interest in her looks was focused on her hair and eyelashes, and the fact that she did not lose her hair during her illness was at least one positive outcome she was grateful to acknowledge. She did not use lipstick or nail varnish, except the latter in later years on her toes to disguise the outcome of my surgical treatment of her ingrown toenails. She suffered from ingrown toenails for most of her adult life. It was the only curable disease she ever had, albeit an ailment that was resistant to treatment in her case. I performed frequent minor surgical procedures on her big toes under local anaesthetic in the comfort of her bedroom. These interventions kept her pain-free and mobile for up to six months at a time. She was very keen to preserve her nails and would only let me do a wedge nail avulsion. She was always delighted with the symptomatic relief and the cosmetic result, though over time, beauty was compromised by repeated surgical insults.

The quid pro quo was that she cut my hair once a month to keep me neat and handsome. This arrangement continued for 30 years. She would pronounce herself very impressed with my surgical skills and forever grateful that she married a surgeon. I, in turn, could not fault her hairdressing talents, which drew admiration and approving glances from my nursing colleagues. The social entrepreneurial economics thus deployed saved me and our private medical insurance company a small fortune, which is now being rapidly recouped by the Pakistani barber in Navan!

Once our children had grown up and left home, Kathleen's social life was as busy as her work life. She managed to play poor golf with willing partners and was an active participant in a regional book club, but above all she loved parties at home and away and, because she had a wide circle of friends, we received many invitations to Dublin. This posed some logistical problems, which we solved by going up to town on the bus and coming home after midnight by taxi. Kathleen was very happy in company – not necessarily mine, although she was always content and safe with me. She enjoyed the buzz of a party and she could walk into a group conversation with easy confidence and aplomb. Better still if she knew those present, but either way, social engagement was natural to her.

I did not mind, as long as she checked on me from time to time to ensure I was not loitering alone at the fringes. I was a reluctant consort, but if she was enjoying the company, I could feign a front. When it came to formal evening functions, Kathleen took it upon herself to handle our seating arrangements: she would first find a seat for me and then take her pick from a number of other invitations before taking her place beside a friendly gentleman colleague.

She was always in demand for house parties and was keen to accept these invitations whenever possible. On the occasions she sensed she was accompanied by a reluctant partner, she would sometimes have a bit of fun at my expense. Usually spurred on by a few extra glasses of wine and playing to any of her male admirers who were present, she would saunter languorously towards wherever I had positioned myself – usually at the exit door ready to chaperone her home.

'What do you think of my legs?' she'd ask me, echoing a constant refrain from our early romantic period, to which it seemed she had never received a satisfactory answer.

'I think they are lovely, Kathleen – now let us get out of here quietly and get a taxi home.'

'No – but what do you *really* think about them?' she'd persist. I'd mumble something suitably racy to keep her happy and gently steer her out. The truth was that by that time the only legs I was interested in were the ones I might have to operate on the next day!

Kathleen had a sixth sense and could detect when I was fully engaging my social skills – in which case, she would come over and quietly ambush me with a six-word admonition: 'Finbar, you are drinking too much!' It was important as a professional couple that the two of us were never both drinking too much at the same time, and I had to be ready and able to utter the same words to her on occasion, much to her annoyance. This was due to the blind spot she had for the variation in wine glass sizes and her misunderstanding of the alcohol volume of certain vintages! Keeping a watchful eye on each other was all part of the contract.

My surgical prowess aside, Kathleen was frequently exasperated at my inability to perform simple household chores and thought I lacked manual dexterity on this front, declaring me 'ham-fisted' at best. Fortunately, however, surgery was not all about simply cutting, knitting and sewing. I was a very good surgeon. I knew what to do and when to do it. How I went about doing it sometimes took longer than necessary, but nobody knew that other than me! I was an old-fashioned surgeon all my working life and, until my retirement and beyond, continued to champion the tried and trusted ways. I never embraced the new technology because I liked to see what I was doing when operating on my patients.

My very good colleague and friend David Bouchier Hayes, who was the great Irish surgical innovator of my day, used to chide me as the 'King Canute' of Irish surgeons. But I knew that keyhole surgery, the greatest technological advance that occurred during my years of practice, was not for me. The 'mirror test' confirmed for me my deficits in hand–eye coordination. I often had difficulty putting on a bow tie in front of a mirror because I could not easily manage to get the T-hook into the eye and would get very frustrated as a result. The T-hook would move in the opposite direction to my hands and I found it very hard to overcome my natural instincts and move my hands in the required way. It is a non-intuitive motor skill that passed me by. Surprisingly, when I turned away from the mirror and could not see, it was easier to do!

For many years, the benefits of keyhole surgery were overstated and thankfully, from my perspective, the transition from open to laparoscopic surgery took some time. My reluctance to change was because I was not happy to depend on a hidden camera in the patient's abdominal cavity to direct me to the diseased organ and to have to fiddle with long-handled hooks and graspers to commence and then carry out the operation. It never made any sense to me and, surprisingly,

I was able to hold back the tide to the end of my service career. These days I also have the added bonus of being able to give a wide berth to formal-dress occasions!

Despite my limitations, I was the resident family surgeon at Greenlawns for 35 years, and I retained my home operating privileges there even after I retired. During my tenure, in addition to the toenail procedures on Mum (her affectionate family name), I performed multiple such operations on Stephen at home and in boarding school, as well as hospital procedures on Peter and Ruth. On one occasion I performed a cosmetic suturing of a peri-orbital laceration on Peter's face; I also did an open appendicectomy on Ruth. All received the seal of approval from Mum and at least modest acknowledgement from our children. Later, however, when Kathleen became ill and was told her cancer was inoperable, the realisation that my surgical skills and experience were redundant and of little benefit to her was a difficult cross to bear, and I felt helpless and lost.

Birthdays and anniversaries were all very important to Kathleen, and successive stepping stones on the horizon of family life throughout the year. They were all pencilled into her diary and imprinted on her mind, a source of joy given and received. I could never keep up with her and she would often chide me for forgetting the children's birthdays, but I celebrated them too. I was just more low-key, whereas she was dancing in the aisles. She celebrated all of these events and occasions, the big and the small, whereas I reserved my dancing for the special ones! She would remind me in advance of them – although I didn't need any pointers as to when each of our babies was on the way.

I always remembered Kathleen's birthday, but she would flag it up to me anyway. It was 20 April, five days before mine. My cards to her were romantic, often with sentimental images and verses, and I'd let them speak for themselves and sign off 'To Kack, with love from Fini'. Her cards were usually contemporary in style and design, and she'd write her greeting theatrically, with a fanfare of pen strokes inviting me to whoop! I'd smile and blow her a kiss, but did not dance. My present would often be one of her favourite chocolate bars or an item of jewellery for which she had a special soft spot. It was a sign to her of my faithful commitment and abiding love – and it always trumped the chocolate! Kathleen's gift to me would be a jumper or jacket, many of which I have had no time to wear. And so, having clothes we'd never worn in our wardrobes was something we had in common.

The births of our four children were another story. Remarkably, perhaps unbelievably, I got through my training years and my entire surgical career without ever witnessing a normal delivery. The closest I got was on the day our third child, Peter, was born. At Kathleen's insistence, and because I hadn't been there for David's or Ruth's arrivals, I was present in the delivery suite at her side as she went into labour. I quickly realised, however, I had picked the wrong birth to attend.

There was a lot of commotion and shuffling of feet around the patient, as the baby decided to take his time descending the canal. Initially I stayed in the wings but soon beat a hasty retreat, feeling that the presence of a watching medic was not conducive to an orderly arrival.

As for the others, I have to report rather shamefacedly that when David was due, in 1980, I was the man who dropped his wife in early labour to Holles Street Hospital and went off to a surgical dinner, only to be summoned when the baby had arrived. Otherwise, Ruth's and Stephen's births were uneventful and, while I was not physically present for either, I was close enough to hear the babies' joyful cries on arrival!

In the later years of our marriage, our love language drifted closer to my end of the spectrum – romantic and sentimental, as per my card choices – as we entered our affectionate, cuddly period. I found the Me to You cards, figurines and bears and we both adopted the associated mascot greeting: 'Me and You / You and Me / That's the way / It'll always be'. The tatty bears and their rhyming refrain kept us company and cheered us up in the good and bad times. After Kathleen's devastating diagnosis and for the time she had left, we would come to rely on these simple words of comfort along with the emojis and our shared humour to assist and sustain us.

7

RETIREMENT AND THE PLEASURES OF LIFE

I often ask myself, why did we do it? Why did we work such rotas and in such conditions, and tolerate them for so long? Because we were so glad to get two jobs back in Ireland at the time and had a young son, and we wanted to be close to the grandparents. Looking for two consultant jobs in the same region in a small country is difficult and involves compromise. Despite the horrors of the rotas, we met some great medical and nursing colleagues and achieved a reasonable amount during our consultant careers.

Since we both retired, I am getting to know Finbar far better. Instead of taking out appendixes, he is taking out weeds and trees from the garden – a bit radically sometimes, I think. That's surgeons for you!

After I retired in early 2012, Kathleen and I spent more time in the garden together. I mowed the seven small lawns, or 'plots' as I called them, and did all the weeding. Kathleen spent her time pottering about with shears and secateurs, pruning and trimming branches, plants and foliage at random. Part of my job was to clean and pick up after her 'garden rounds'. I always got praise for my gardening activities, and in retirement I increased my workload to please her more – and myself. She continued to work in the hospital in Navan for another two years after my retirement. I did more of the simple domestic shopping and cooking (nothing fancy) and looked forward to her coming home in the evenings to share all the hospital news. She was more keen to discuss her projects in the medical unit and the developments she had championed now that I was a 'has-been' and thus more able to give her unbiased commentary and advice. On many occasions she would arrive home with her car full of colour and vegetation, which signalled garden business only. She would summon me to unload the boot and then to dig holes to bury the bulbs and plant the flowers. There was no grand plan and anywhere would do. We lived in a ramshackle house, and so it was fitting we should also have such a garden.

I had always been able to unwind after a long day's work in the hospital by spending time on my weeding duties and, once every two weeks, cutting the lawns with my push-mower. 'You are a great boy, Dad,' Kathleen would remark when I brought my labours to her attention. Weeding was usually safe from censure as her eyes were focused only on the plants and flowers.

After our separate days in our respective hospitals, we'd manage to work happily together in the garden.

When I retired, the garden became my operating theatre. Much of my new approach to the work followed spur-of-the-moment decisions, and no tree, plant or flower was safe from surgical extinction! The feeling of joy and fulfilment on removing, chopping or excising large chunks of wood and vegetation in one fell swoop was exhilarating and spurred me on to make an impression before Kathleen arrived home. When she returned to inspect the work performed to please her, she always feared the worst.

'That's not a weed, Finbar, that's one of my hydrangeas!' I knew I was in trouble when she addressed me by my Christian name.

'Well, it looks like a weed,' was my lame excuse.

'If you are not sure, don't touch it without asking me.' As a reply, it was a real comedown for a surgeon …

It was only then that I realised that the weeds were mine and everything else in the garden was hers!

While Kathleen continued working at the hospital, I needed some mental sustenance to keep me sane and it came in the form of student teaching. When I was not in the garden with the weeds, I was in the hospital with the medical students. They were fun to be with yet kept me on my toes. I had to keep up with all the new developments in surgery and could not rely on the old-fashioned didactic teaching methods to survive but had to engage them in interactive discussion and answer their questions. It was a privilege and a rewarding opportunity to pass on my experiences and insights.

And so, as well as my gardening activities, my routine in retirement has included my twice-weekly teaching sessions on the wards of the Mater. Every Tuesday and Wednesday morning during term times, I catch the 6.40 a.m. bus from Collon to Dublin, having been briefed on the Monday evening about suitable teaching cases by the surgical tutor attached to the hospital's professorial unit.

Now that I am retired, I always wear an identity badge when giving my bedside tutorials. When I was in active practice, everybody in the hospital knew who I was, but now I need the badge to gain access to the wards. Often I need to present it for close inspection to the nurses and patients before I can engage and set about organising the teaching sessions – only then do they acknowledge my status. The students are easily recognised by their white coats but they also wear larger badges with their first names in bold print for ease of recognition. They go around in pairs or threesomes with a visible air of excitement at being on the wards at last and experiencing at first hand the hustle and bustle of hospital medicine. They are all attached to different surgical teams and spend most of their time attending clinics, operating sessions and ward rounds. They stare eagerly at the patients from a distance, looking out for signs that they have permission to approach, whereas my own searching clinical gaze from a distance is first seeking to identify suitable patients for my teaching session. If my smile is acknowledged and reciprocated by a patient, I can generally assume that I have captured a willing subject for the tutorial! I introduce myself and explain the teaching procedure and seek the patient's consent to be a participant. Most are happy to help. The students enjoy the bedside tutorials because they get a chance to take a patient's history and present it to their colleagues, and then I intervene to reveal the gaps in their knowledge. They tend to accept my put-downs with grace and will focus on regrouping themselves for next time.

The history, or story, of the illness as recounted by the patient to the student can be a riveting revelation. When the patient is a good historian and able to give a concise account with the most pertinent details of their case, the diagnosis will generally be obvious and easy to discern, resulting in an early win for the well-prepared student. Equally, however, a history recounted by a patient who is a rambler may appear unpredictable and baffling, leaving the student, no matter how clever, completely stumped. In the early days of term they are mostly stumped anyway, not only by the patients' use of the vernacular and, in some cases, their accents, but also by the difficulty of adapting to a new learning experience as they transition from medical theory to practice.

I suspect that my interjections, advice and direction are usually forgotten before the day has passed, but here goes, one more time:

'If they have a story, let them tell it without interruption. Leading questions are often unsettling for the patient and tend to upset the normal flow. If the history is going off-track, let it go where it wants for a time. It may appear to be a weird journey and full of loose ends. Medical stories are not always neat and tidy, and often you have to start again on a different track.

'Whenever they were last well is the start of the illness. Coming to hospital by ambulance is an acute presentation, whereas coming to the clinic is usually a non-urgent or elective case.

'The only information you need about pain is about its onset and where and how severe it is. If you ask too many questions about a single symptom, you will get lost and confused. If a patient's presenting complaint is abdominal pain, the problem is most often surgical. Which system is the patient complaining about? Listen for clues. If he or she has indigestion, nausea or vomiting, it is either gullet, stomach, gallbladder or upper gut. If there is blood in the toilet bowl, it is gut, bladder or kidney. If the skin is yellow, it is gallbladder, liver or pancreas. If you are still unsure, ask the patient what the diagnosis is. They often know and are always happy to tell you. Even if they are unsure, they may have been told the test results, and if so, they may be able to give you some useful clues, providing you know the correct follow-up questions to ask. If the patient does not know, it may be that the diagnosis is not established yet.'

My bedside tutorials, the patients and the students would be a sometimes unsettling counterpoint for me during Kathleen's illness and, after she died, a source of rescue and repair. A hospital ward initially felt like a surprising space for grieving and for trying to understand and come to terms with a mysterious and unknown illness. In time, it has become a kind of home for me, one I share with a group of trustworthy souls and where I have some sense of control.

❖

In 2014, at the age of 65, I retired from my HSE public hospital job in Navan. The hospital hosted a 60s-themed 'rock and roll' party in the Navan O'Mahony's GAA park, and I was presented with a ceremonial cake shaped like a cardiac defibrillator. I felt very nostalgic, leaving the hospital and all my wonderful friends after all those years, but also a little relieved to relinquish the stresses of providing an acute medical service in those days of 'trolley medicine' [the practice whereby patients must wait on trolleys for their medical treatment], inadequate resources and increasing patient expectations.

After my retirement, I continued to work part-time in the Mater Private Outreach Clinic in the town. I started to think more about our four children and how they were going to fare. Ruth was now married but there was no sign of any long-term romantic prospects for any of the boys.

The garden had always been a happy place for us to unwind after long days at work. In later years, it was where we were best able to reflect on our life together and where our children were heading, as well as to exchange sweet nothings to affirm our loving companionship.

'I wonder, Dad, should we have sent them to day school? Were we thinking more of ourselves?'

'I don't know, Mum, but I think it has worked out OK for them. They have good friends from schooldays and have grown up fast.'

After a momentary pause for effect, she said, 'All the McGarrys went to day school and all the Lennons went to boarding school.'

She was referring to our own generation but was making a subtle observation about the new Lennon generation, all of whom had also gone to boarding school. I knew I was not going to win this joust and decided to attempt a strategic retreat and hold my own counsel. I could often read her mind, which on this occasion, I realised, was pondering why none of the children had done Medicine. Yes, we both would have liked one of them to follow the path we had taken, but that was another matter. Kathleen did not tend to linger on this topic and quickly moved on, but it did nag her at times.

Maybe our professional lives defined us for the children. Perhaps we were not well-rounded role models. We were both busy doctors engaged exclusively in the sciences and had little time for the humanities, akin to 'all work and no play'. We were unable to give them sufficient protected time with us separately and together. Kathleen was more aware of this and was far better at time management than me. She made great efforts to get the balance right and I believe she did so in her engagement with each of them, while I was trailing far behind. The growth of their individual personalities took place against this backdrop. Each was different but perhaps they had needed more from us together. Even my periodic flights into poetry were generally greeted with groans rather than as some kind of source of inspiration!

It was after one such 'garden round' conversation with Kathleen that I penned a short poem that was a wistful reflection on longed-for milestones not yet in sight and alluded to our advancing years, the fact that none of our four grown-up children was married as yet and that grandchildren were still a distant prospect:

We fed the bulbs to tangled sod
Sideways or upright did not matter.
Wan winter sunlight just reached the spot
We chose to start another cycle.
Our modest milestones ticked for 2012
But failing time the enemy beside.
The landscape trembling cold
And the dull sameness on the horizon.

A glazed gaze on gnarled rural pastures
Now forlorn for want of renewal.
The energy of young fitful steps
Missing for two old friends.
Setting the clock back to slow the time
Gives some relief.
But will it be enough?

All parents look forward to becoming grannies and grandads. It's a second coming: an opportunity to join a new junior team and don the jersey again, redress past mistakes and attempt to fulfil the 'super-parent' role with enhanced results under less pressure. It does not always work out, but at least you are no longer indispensable. Kathleen's parents had relished their roles as grandparents to our children, as had mine. My father was a doting grandad, and Granny Lennon followed his example and very much enjoyed getting to know David and Ruth (sadly, she died before she would have the opportunity to meet either Peter or Stephen). Like 'Granny Garry', she was an English teacher and was responsible for my initial interest in literature.

Kathleen continued to be bemused by the Lennon family dynamic, which she remarked on from time to time in the course of the more prolonged garden chats of our retirement.

'I cannot understand how you have never been to your sisters' houses in Lincoln and Southampton,' was a frequent admonishment.

'Well, Mum, I *have* been to Southampton once!'

I have noticed since she died that I have become more like her, so she must have passed something on to me in our many years together. I was always sentimental but my newly acquired traits include softness, a greater capacity for acceptance, and patience. It's a good mix and I am all the better for it.

❖

My involvement with the Irish Heart Foundation has been a joy and I believe I have contributed to its advancement in a positive way. I was also delighted to have played a role in the development of the Royal College of Physicians in Ireland and to have been a voice for colleagues in the smaller hospitals and to advocate for important issues relating to women in medicine. I was very fortunate to be well enough to carry out my professional management role in the Royal College of Physicians in Ireland (RCPI). This sense of still being useful is so important to my own self-worth.

I was interviewed at the European Society of Cardiology's Annual Congress in 2015 and asked what advice I give to young cardiologists. I tell them that cardiology is a very satisfying career that offers infinite variety. There are very few other fields that provide such a range of options. You can specialise in invasive cardiology, echocardiography, preventive cardiology or even, for those who like research, go down the academic route. As you go through the training programme, you're likely to find that one element stands out for you above all others. Young people also need to be assertive in lobbying training bodies to make trainee schemes more family friendly by offering more flexible part-time training and job sharing. This is particularly important bearing in mind that over 50 per cent of the medical workforce are women.

When Kathleen retired from hospital practice in Navan, she devoted more of her time to her professional college, the Royal College of Physicians in Ireland (RCPI) and the Irish Heart Foundation (IHF). She already had a long association with both and was keen to serve and assist them in promoting their key aims. She was well respected and was a very open and sympathetic colleague, who was able to navigate the world of medical politics with ease, and she had no agenda. Her significant contribution to medical practice in Ireland was widely acknowledged by her peers. She was appointed President of the IHF and took on this role as it was about to celebrate its 50th anniversary in 2016; she was its first female president. The vision and purpose of the IHF was to ensure people in Ireland live more active, healthy lives, free from heart disease and stroke. Kathleen was in the vanguard of promoting its vision and strategy during her short term in office.

At the same time, she took on a busy executive role in the RCPI. The College was her second home and she enjoyed the company of physician colleagues which she had missed during most of her working life in Navan. She was a constant presence on its council for 25 years, being consistently re-elected every two years by her colleagues. In her earlier days, she was often the only woman on the ballot paper and so, as there were only a relatively small number of female voters, she was dependent on the men for support! However, it was universally acknowledged within the College that she was chosen each time on merit. She looked forward to the bi-monthly council meetings and was an active participant in all its deliberations. Her perspective on the issues of the day was sought and valued, and her experience and consensus approach gave her currency and credibility. She was a consistent and dedicated advocate for female medics and particularly for trainee doctors. She enjoyed the occasional formal dignified spat at council meetings with some of her 'cognitive physician' colleagues. Her impish sense of humour was often on display at informal meetings, receptions and dinners, and never did her any harm!

Over the years Kathleen made two unsuccessful attempts to become president of the College and, while disappointed to lose out, she was glad each time that she 'put her hat in the ring'. She would often remark on the large portraits of the male presidents lined up on the historic walls and staircases of the College. She was always looking and hoping that one day there would be a portrait of a woman president among their ranks. And so she was delighted when in 2017, the College fellows elected Dr Mary Horgan as RCPI's first female President. In the final analysis Kathleen was very happy to have been a wise and reliable colleague who was appreciated and valued by her peers.

PART TWO

8

DIAGNOSIS

For most of my life I had suffered from what we medics call upper gastrointestinal dyspepsia, so-called 'indigestion'. I had telescope tests (OGDs) and CT scans. The diagnosis was always non-specific gastritis and I was prescribed antacids (PPIs), which I continued to take for over 25 years. In addition I suffered from diverticulitis [inflammation in pockets of the large bowel causing severe pain in the lower abdomen] and was admitted to hospital on three occasions, in one instance under the care of my husband! Aside from this, I had two operations, one to have my gallbladder removed and another to remove a benign ovarian cyst.

Around Christmas 2015, my indigestion symptoms became troublesome again and my epigastric and left flank pain was more constant. I decided to have another OGD. This again revealed some gastritis which was biopsied but did not reveal any significant pathology. However my conscientious physician at the time decided to arrange a CT scan of my abdomen. The scan revealed a number of moderately enlarged glands behind my stomach ('retroperitoneal nodes'). This was potentially a worrisome finding but was not specific, and the advice was to wait and repeat the scan in three months. In the meantime I had a PET scan which is more sensitive in picking up cancer disease and this test came back 'normal'. My symptoms settled on antacids for a time, and I forgot about my troubles.

The repeat CT scan three months later showed the glands had increased in size and number. I was shocked and very worried, and began to realise this was not going to work out well. My consultant CO'M [Colm O'Morain] arranged a biopsy which was performed on 25 April, Finbar's birthday.

Two days later, on 27 April 2016, I got my cancer diagnosis.

The surprising thing was that Kathleen looked the picture of health. She had a lot of benign symptoms that seemed to be more of a nuisance than a menace. Indigestion in all its forms, migraine headaches and restless legs were lifelong ailments for her, which flared up from time to time. She took them in her stride. It was only when the pattern and frequency of some of her abdominal symptoms changed that her 'medical brain' grew increasingly worried and upset. She was more aware of her symptoms at night. This is, of course, the time the senses express themselves to greatest effect and, in return, receive the most attention. The distractions of the busy day over, the mind's focus turns to the woes of the body, which seem magnified, sometimes out of all proportion. In the darkness, there is no objective means to hand to manage the wandering anxiety and distress of the sleepless patient. Medicines provide some transient relief but only dull the senses. Pain, the main signal of Kathleen's illness, became a constant night-time bedfellow and then spilled into the day. It is the symptom that is often the most difficult to control and one that is always suffered alone.

When accessing medical care here in Ireland, the patient's first port of call is nearly always the general practitioner (GP), or family doctor, who in turn will refer onwards those patients requiring specialist advice or intervention. This referral pattern has changed somewhat due to Google, and some patients are now bypassing the family doctor and seeking out consultant specialists at the outset. Once you attend the family doctor or hospital by appointment, you become a patient. Doctors with a real or imagined illness will often try every trick to avoid that label for themselves. For those outside the medical profession, this might seem hard to understand – after all, don't we have confidence that our colleagues can treat us; and why would we imagine that we would be exempt from health problems, which are part of the human condition?

But the truth is that when doctors fall ill their sense of vulnerability is all the greater because of the sudden, unaccustomed reversal of roles that takes place – from always being in control to a state of submission. Suddenly they see their hard-won cherished world of benevolent power spiralling away and are hopelessly lost in the crowd. It feels better for the doctor-patient to take a leaf from the Bible and retain autonomy by applying the exhortation, 'Physician, heal thyself', and simply hoping that things will work out for them.

Kathleen informally discussed her indigestion symptoms with a family-doctor friend, who filled out her prescriptions for antacid medications, but then went her own way and only opted to take the conventional medical triage route late in the day. This was not surprising, as she was a general medical consultant who tended to self-diagnose and medicate, and only when she was unable to cure herself did she decide to self-refer to a consultant colleague. For most of her life, she believed – unwisely – that she had no need for either of the above medical resources, GP or consultant. This was perhaps doubly unwise in a family where both parents were carriers of an abnormal gene associated with Factor 5 Leiden Deficiency (a condition where there is an increased risk of developing abnormal blood clots), which caused DVTs in both of us and in Ruth and subsequent pulmonary emboli (clotting in the lungs) in two of us. In addition to this, both Kathleen and I suffered from inflammatory bowel disease, as does one of our children, while another has seronegative arthritis (a form of rheumatoid arthritis). Kathleen provided treatment options for all of us, and she kept a well-stocked pharmacy of medications for that purpose.

Despite her somewhat unconventional management of her own medical complaints and symptoms, her philosophy was to do everything possible to stay healthy. In her professional life, she embraced the old motto of 'prevention is better than cure' and was a passionate advocate for that approach during her long association with the IHF. In this sense, she was always careful about her own health and had regular check-ups. She never missed her breast-screening appointments or her annual reviews with her gynaecologist and made frequent visits to the dentist because she did not want to lose her teeth in later years. And because of her long-standing indigestion, she had had many OGD examinations over the years, following self-referral to gastroenterology colleagues. One of the stigmas associated with cancer is that it is somehow your fault – and while certain deliberate behaviours (such as smoking and drinking alcohol to excess) can be contributory factors, even then this stigma and its subliminal inference is hurtful and depressing and leaves you feeling very isolated. In her case, she did not have this additional psychological cross to bear, as she could not have done much more to avoid the malady or to have had it detected at an early or pre-invasive stage.

If Kathleen was an advocate of the preventive approach when it came to her own care, I was the opposite. I was afraid of health checks for fear that something would turn up! I only attended the doctor when something was wrong, even though Kathleen did push me to have occasional bowel checks because of my history of inflammatory bowel disease. In my defence, I was very much aware of the growing emphasis in medicine on carrying out multiple tests and investigations, not only on sick patients but, worryingly, also on healthy ones. There is a resultant risk, particularly with X-rays such as CT scans, of incidental findings being picked up that are not necessarily important but may cause the patient a great deal of extra anxiety and stress. In such instances, I always explained that a finding that was unrelated to the presenting complaint was not significant, and I would reassure the patient. I suppose I never considered that my unequivocal opinion might not always have been correct or that the patient might not agree with my analysis.

When Kathleen was told she had a number of enlarged glands that were probably incidental, she was worried and not totally convinced of their innocence, but I was happy to accept the doctor's reassurance, even though it was not as unequivocal as mine usually was. After all, she had none of the clinical signs of illness that I'd always relied on in my practice to alert me to the possibility of underlying disease. In addition, her parents had lived into their early 90s and she had been vigilant about her health. So she had no reason to fear the relatively early onset of a devastating illness. That was why I found it so difficult to believe at first, although, from the moment the enlarged glands were noted to have increased in size and number, we knew a cancer diagnosis was a possibility. We had not considered that before because she was so well.

I recall visiting a surgical colleague to discuss the findings of the follow-up CT scan, and his opinion was that, as the only abnormality found on imaging was enlarged para-aortic glands, it was more likely that she had a lymphoma, which is potentially curable. I did my best to reassure Kathleen that if it was a cancer, it could be successfully treated. I reminded her that we both had relatives and friends who had been treated for various cancers and were now well. And so we were ready to face the music with fortitude and resolve, along with some degree of confidence and hope that this was a manageable situation.

9

MOMENT OF IMPACT

Wednesday, 27 April 2016

a.m.: Cancer – I have it. Call at 9:30 from CO'M, my consultant: 'We have to talk about this. Can you come today? Will Finbar come? No, it is not lymphoma. They don't know the source.' Sounds bad. I read in the Irish Independent *newspaper on Monday about Dermot Morgan's [the actor who played Father Ted] young son, Ben, who was recently diagnosed with Nodular Sclerosing Hodgkin's Disease and had started writing a blog about his experience which has helped him ... I'll see. Feel sick. Finbar examining in Final Med. in Mater. Text him to ring me. Cancel my afternoon Mater Clinic in Navan. Go to Beacon Clinic to hear the worst.*

p.m.: CO'M tells us its metastatic AdenoCa [adenocarcinoma]. GI? Ovarian? Obviously great shock for CO'M. We are shattered. We don't know source. Further histology required. Colonoscopy in a.m. Up all night with the lovely drinks!

He did not just say it was cancer. He knew he had to be more precise and to quickly give us all the information about the test results because we were medical colleagues. In the circumstances, the opportunity to break the news gently and incrementally was not an option. Everything about the diagnosis was bad. He had to be candid, and it was best to get it over with and tell us all. In the event, he managed to be candid, gentle and kind all at once.

We listened in silence and between us picked up most of what he had to say. He told us the biopsy confirmed metastatic adenocarcinoma but said that they were unable to determine the source of the disease, or what is called the 'primary site', and that sometimes this is never found. I knew immediately this diagnosis was on the other end of the scale to a lymphoma. There were no silver linings to cling to for comfort. All the trappings of medical status, knowledge and security drained away, as we were confronted with an unknown advanced cancer. At that moment we both knew the odds were stacked against us. Questions crowded our minds but there was little point in asking them at the time. I don't know exactly how to describe it. It was like a car crash, and the moment of impact was life-changing. We left Colm O'Morain's office in a daze with our emotions locked in neutral. Her years of chronic gastritis had been replaced overnight with terminal cancer. For both of us, it was as stark as that, yet the only way to manage was to pretend it was not the case. The key dilemma for us was that at the time she was fully involved in the routine of family and professional life. Should she stop or go?

This contradiction – between knowing what the diagnosis meant and needing to act as if things were otherwise, just to be able to carry on – would lie at the heart of everything we said and did from this point onwards and throughout almost the entire course of Kathleen's illness.

> *I had been practising medicine as a consultant physician for 32 years and had never come across a case like mine. The news was broken to me by my physician colleague and friend who was also a classmate. He was as devastated by the news as I was. He told me the only treatment was chemotherapy and that, as I was in good physical condition, I should be able to tolerate it. I constantly ask myself how come I have this advanced cancer, with two such healthy parents. Fortunately my mother died without the anxiety of knowing about my disease.*

The transition from being two doctors in full control of our patients' destinies to becoming lost and helpless souls in an instant was a numbing experience – the more so because there was no treatment map to tackle this unknown killer. How to cope, manage and survive consumed our thoughts on the silent journey home that day. My duty was to fight the bleak sentence that had been handed down with all my strength, knowledge and experience and, more importantly, to constantly reassure

Kathleen that all was not lost. She was now a patient but it was important I did not become one too.

Once home, we had to prepare for the next day. She started drinking the bowel-stimulating laxative fluid, and the diarrhoea commenced around midnight. Neither of us slept that night. She spent the night running from her room to the toilet, while I lay awake in the adjoining room, waiting to get up in time the next morning and occasionally checking in with her to murmur words of encouragement and support.

Thursday, 28 April 2016
Colonoscopy in Beacon; two small polyps excised, but not the source.

Met our son Stephen in Beacon. The news is too much for me. Still on autopilot. Finbar great support. We have to await further detailed histology results before hopefully identifying source. Have URTI [upper respiratory tract infection]. Now inclined to think everything is related to diagnosis. We have to stay positive.

We cannot decide which hospital to go to for Oncology.

Children phoned. Ruth 18 weeks pregnant – great news. Don't want to upset her. Thoughts – Ruth's baby due in October: first grandchild. Will I see? Decided with Finbar to attend Professor DC [Des Carney] in the Mater. Finbar has worked with him for years, an experienced and sensible oncologist.

Colm O'Morain had reassured us that the diagnosis could not have been made earlier as, apart from her indigestion, which had been investigated by regular endoscopy examinations, she had no other significant complaints and was otherwise healthy and clinically well. He kindly agreed to contact the oncologist and provide him with a summary of her case.

Friday, 29 April 2016
Had Mammogram. Normal.
I remember going into the Breast Unit in the Mater Hospital and meeting a colleague radiologist there, and telling her she was unlikely to have ever come across a patient who fervently hoped she would be diagnosed with breast cancer, but that is how I felt on the day, knowing I could cope with a cancer disease that had a name. Finbar met pathologist in Beaumont hospital to discuss histology results.

Saturday, 30 April 2016
All children down home for weekend. Finbar put file together with all information to give to the oncologist, DC.

Tuesday, 3 May 2016
Met Professor DC who had reviewed histology report. I had previously had bilateral oophorectomy [surgical removal of both ovaries] for benign ovarian cysts in 2014. That ruled out ovarian cancer. That left upper GI as likely source, possibly stomach or pancreas. We were told all relevant tests had been

done and that further testing was pointless. DC advised that I should start chemotherapy.

A few days after we were given the diagnosis, I went to visit the pathologist, a friend of mine. I remember sitting down with her and peering into the microscope to view the rogue cells. They did not look remarkable to me, and I recall her gently explaining the abnormal features on the apparently harmless slides.

'Finbar, the cells from the biopsy are adenocarcinoma cells and we have done further immunochemistry tests on the sample. That information suggests the primary could be in the gut, more likely in the upper part, or the pancreas. Other possible – less likely – sites are ovary, breast and lung.'

I nodded in acknowledgement but remained silent. She seemed anxious to ensure I could recognise the problem, but even at my best, she was assuming a knowledge base in pathology that was beyond me. It was a surreal experience. I thanked her for her kindness and collegial support and she hugged me as I left her office.

The immediate post-diagnosis days were filled with more tests and car journeys; the evenings with unanswered questions punctuating long silent periods as we both busied ourselves performing routine household chores, hers purposeful and mine pointless. We were both grappling separately with our hopes and fears, trying to make sense of it all. During those days Kathleen often asked me all the questions that were whirring about her mind, to which I had no answers. 'Well, what do you think, Dad?' 'How could this happen?' 'What did I do wrong?' 'What are we going to do?' She was intentionally leaving the questions hanging in the air and not developing her line of thought. Her sister Joan often referred to Kathleen's habit of opening a conversation with the word 'Well', followed by a pause. It was an opening gambit that facilitated the delivery of good or bad news, and a subtle invitation to the other person to respond first, so that his or her disposition could be determined. I am fond of non sequiturs and frequently use the device in conversation and, though not as subtle as Kathleen's strategy, I find this is also a way of buying time to frame a response.

'Maybe, Mum, I should get the front plot done before it rains.' She was happy enough with that retort. I knew she did not really want me to answer the questions just then.

10

CANDLES AND PRAYERS

Why are there so many prayer books for the dying? I want a prayer book for getting better. I have my medal of Our Lady of Perpetual Succour, but I wonder about God. I hate the way they call us 'sinners' in all the prayers, and all the fire and brimstone they go on about. Will the Masses being said for my intentions be of any use, or the Novenas, or the Shrines or the Scapulars? My holy friends, including my housekeeper, tell me about the prayer meetings and the retreats and how important they are. I hope there is something in it. Must read up the evidence.

I remember how, when I was a young boy in the 1950s, we always looked forward to a big Church event or feast day like the Corpus Christi procession or the midnight Masses at Christmas and Easter. They always pulled in the crowds, and all prayers for personal intentions were welcomed for consideration by the saints. Now, in more recent times, cancer in its own perverse way is drawing in the crowds with a promise of relief and a reasonable expectation of a cure in many cases. There is no longer mention of the Church in the treatment plan, with so many medical advances having occurred over the last 50 years. Well into my reflective years, I wondered how relevant the Church was now, as Kathleen embarked on this last journey. The Church wants us to believe that sickness, health and faith are constant partners and that each lives beside and serves the other. If the medicine does not work, what are the alternative options, if any? What about prayer, or is it just preparing you for the end? Can prayer, which seemed to work long ago, still lead to a cure? If not, can it assist and provide some comfort and solace?

If medicine does not cure you, it seems unlikely prayer will. But I suppose you have to try it first, and of course you can continue to pray long after medicine has run its course. And prayer is not dependent on evidence! When we first got the news of Kathleen's diagnosis, we realised that other options apart from medicine had to figure in our 'survival plan'. We were both Sunday Mass goers and retained some of the faith of our fathers and mothers. I had believed in the spiritual power of candles since I was a child, though the evidence base is pretty weak. I remember lighting seven candles with a flame in Dublin's Pro-Cathedral the day before her biopsy report came through and praying for a good test result for her. On that occasion it failed me. At the time she was not convinced about prayers or candles and I recall her sister Pat telling her, 'All prayers are answered, though not always in the way we want,' to which Kathleen's response was, 'Even if you are well-off?'

Candles are lit for prayer intentions and a donation box is located beside the candle rack. A statue with a candle prayer reading is close by – for example, 'Virgin Mother, I place in your care the intention for which I light this candle.' It seems important to light a candle with a flame. For me, these votive candles are more authentic than the newer light-bulb candles that you just switch on. The cost of candles – or the 'offering' as it is called – is usually posted on the candle rack and its purpose is simply to defray expenses. The guidance cost can range from as little as 10 cents in churches in poor areas of the city up to 80 cents in the more affluent suburbs. Perhaps it would be more appropriate if no such guidance was given, as the Catholic ethos does not discriminate between rich and poor, and if the intention is pure, any offering, no matter how small or large, should be accepted with gratitude.

I probably qualify as an occasional pilgrim or penitent, since I belong more to the secular than the spiritual world. In times of need or distress, I often turn to God, but it is very easy to unwittingly behave in a secular way or to wear 'two hats'! If I am seeking a big or special favour, I will of my own volition consider lighting additional candles or paying a higher sum. This potentially renders any spiritual interaction null and void, as the transaction becomes 'commercial', even though it is private and is not recorded or formally acknowledged. My faults and failings in this regard are facilitated by the Church authorities, who do not need to place a value on the offering. The solidarity between rich and poor will always cover expenses, but it is generally the poor who fill the boxes and pay more.

There may be some spiritual rationale for this practice of giving guidance costs, as the Church may wish to challenge the penitent's bona fides. The customary leaving of an offering provides the opportunity for a fascinating subjective examination of one's disposition and motives, because the likely response to the request for spiritual intervention, if there is any, will surely be determined by the purity of one's actions. Buying forgiveness, or ensuring the intercession of the angels and saints (some of whom, like doctors, have specialty interests) against disease or poor health through the donation of money was always an interesting if dubious proposition, even though the motives of the unwitting supplicants are often genuine.

My own candle activity, which had been ongoing for many years, stems from my sincere belief in the practice and was generally directed at seeking good health for my wife and four children, as well as lighting an extra one or two for a friend in need. I continue to believe that lighting a candle is a re-enactment of some element of the faith I was taught in school.

Our housekeeper, Rosemary, is a very devout Catholic who believes in the power of prayer, and on hearing the news of Kathleen's illness, she immediately sprang into action. Within a short space of time, she had placed a banner icon on the kitchen table, instructing me to pray in front of it for seven consecutive days, which I did. Meanwhile, she had special Masses said for our intentions in all the local churches, and friends and nursing colleagues of Kathleen did likewise.

There was a renewed fervour to my prayers, and though neither of us became more devout – initially, in any case – we did continue with our normal Catholic obligations. We felt happy and blessed that many of our new friends became so devout on our behalf. I also felt very fortunate to have a second special devout Catholic friend, whom I met regularly at early-morning Mass in Berkeley Road Church opposite the Mater Hospital. Theresa is a daily early-morning Mass goer and saw a halo around my head from day one! She was always accompanied by one of her septuagenarian brothers, Paddy or Leo, and sometimes by both, if Leo had been able to rise at 7 a.m. Theresa has a great memory and any family information I shared was retained. She followed Kathleen's journey with sadness and gentle, caring kindness. She was also a good source of income for the church because she lit candles every morning and outscored me in her tally each time!

11

PREPARING FOR TREATMENT

7–8 May 2016

We went away for the weekend to Rathmullan in Donegal, one of our favourite holiday spots, where we used to bring the children at Easter time when they were very young. We walked hand-in-hand on the strand in front of the hotel. We went to a healing Mass in Oughterlin, just outside the village. On our way home, we stopped in Ardee Golf Club. Finbar gave me the new 'driver' he had bought for my birthday and I hit some golf balls on the range. I did not get a chance to use it again.

On 10 May I was admitted to MPH [Mater Private Hospital] for insertion of the access port for infusion of the chemotherapy. The procedure went well. Finbar and I met DC again next day, and he discussed the chemo regime of Oxaliplatin, 5FU and Leucovorin. I was told it involved wearing an infusion pump at home after every chemo session for 48 hours in a special over-the-shoulder bag.

To prepare myself for treatment, I went with my two sisters, Pat and Joan, to The Hair Club shop in Donnybrook. I bought a full wig, which reminded me of my hair in the 70s when I was a student. I also got a wonderful clip-on hairpiece for top and sides. This all turned out to be a great success, to the extent that people would say, 'And your hair never fell out!' My hair thinned rather than fell out and the hairpiece disguised this well. My eyebrows and eyelashes remained unaffected, to my amazement. This was a great boost for me as it enabled me to continue many of my jobs with some confidence.

When Kathleen and I commenced practice in Ireland in the 1980s, the protocol for dealing with patients with cancer was different from today. Then, the clinician who made the cancer diagnosis would oversee the management of the case, even though multiple specialty disciplines were involved in the patient's care. This is no longer the case, and for most cancer patients now, particularly those with metastatic cancer, the primary treating consultant will be the oncologist. I am not sure this is always in the best interest of the patient. This is not a criticism of oncologists but, by definition, their focus and perspective are very much on the cancer disease. When it is metastatic, the horse has bolted, so to speak, and chemotherapy at best may slow its progress but, in truth, it is often little more than palliative treatment at that stage. The loss of autonomy and sense of shock for the patient is often profound and many patients require additional time, attention, space and reassurance to come to terms with the illness. The general practitioner or generalist physician is best placed to provide this kind of support, and in retrospect it was unfortunate that resource was not there for Kathleen from the outset. That was our own fault because we chose to bypass the GP route – a common response in a profession that often does not practise what it preaches!

If there is any hope of cure, the cancer patient who is 'well' will take his or her chances with any treatment option and the doctor-turned-patient is no different. We knew that surgery offers the best treatment for the management of a solid cancer and that chemotherapy and radiotherapy are complementary add-ons that work best when the diseased tissue, or most of it, has been surgically removed. In a case such as Kathleen's, where the primary disease is unknown and where the surgical route is therefore not an option, there is no evidence that chemo- or radiotherapy are of much benefit, although they may on some occasions add a few months to the survival time. Whereas I understood this clinical dilemma, or thought I did, we were doubly disadvantaged because as doctors we were very aware of the likely course of the disease, and its bleak prognosis. We had an excellent, caring oncologist whom we knew and trusted, but the wheels had come off and we were lost.

Cancer is a common disease and is increasing in frequency. Once you have been diagnosed with it, it's too late to ask why you got it, so that avenue of discourse, while inevitable, is not productive. If it is an early cancer and is localised, it can be cured or managed as a chronic illness. In that case it is often possible to resume a near-normal life. If it is an advanced cancer, your mission suddenly becomes one of how to make the best of what time is left. Yes, you can factor a cure or a miracle into your prayers – when Kathleen's diagnosis was confirmed, various colleagues and friends recounted stories to us of people with advanced cancers who beat the odds and remained well for years down the road. You feign optimism and surprise in order to acknowledge their kindly wishes, but know you have no choice but to don a suit of armour and hope you have the strength of purpose to soldier on.

You get a lot of advice about chemo before you start the treatment and most of it is preparing you for trouble. Kathleen's oncologist's take on her treatment prospects was positive, tempered with a measure of caution. Though there were undoubted caveats in the 'terms and conditions', there were no doom-and-gloom moments in his presentation of the situation. His glass was half-full, and we were relieved we could at least assume a modestly upbeat disposition.

Kathleen then had two information sessions with the oncology nurses. Most of the details she received from them was about the side-effects of chemo and how to manage them.

The list of side-effects was long and she was warned she would suffer some or all of them. Little information was provided about its complementary, potentially positive impact on the disease. For the cancers it cures, the risk–benefit ratio is always acceptable, but for the bad cancers, it is a much more difficult call. Kathleen's case was at the wrong end of the spectrum, and though the nurses were upbeat and kind, their glass was clearly half-empty.

There is a fascinating dynamic between the consultant and the specialty nurse that I had observed in my own practice. As a surgeon, I was on a much sounder footing than the oncologist because I could propose removing the cancer and hold the evidence in my hands. I spent most of my time in practice explaining and talking up the benefits of surgery: its potential to cure, its ability to at least improve the patient's quality of life. After I'd had my say, the nurse had to modify or manage the elevated expectations of the patient and inform them about the downsides and detailed side-effects of treatment.

Over the years, I saw many patients with advanced cancers and always encouraged them not to be frightened or despondent. However, now that my wife was on the receiving end of a diagnosis of an advanced cancer with no known primary, I realised that my professional, reassuring approach may on occasions have been misplaced and unwise. For two experienced doctors in our situation, adopting such a positive and upbeat attitude at the outset was foolish and had to be binned.

We had just entered a dark cul-de-sac and, to my alarm, Kathleen already knew how poor the prognosis was and that the years ahead had become months. I spent a lot of time researching the literature in those early days, and it became very clear that there is no treatment for metastatic adenocarcinoma of unknown origin. The time left is set, no matter how well you feel. Chemotherapy is not going to cure you. It is simply a crutch to lean on for a while. The good days you now enjoy will be reduced by half once the treatment commences, yet the number of days left will stay the same. That's what I learned with a heavy heart, but I knew I had to bury that knowledge and somehow adopt a completely contrary position.

It meant tapping into the virtue of hope and instilling it into all our deliberations. We already had a deep emotional attachment and my role was to address Kathleen's fears by using every personal and social encounter to make her feel safe. To my surprise and relief, I was able to do so, and from the beginning, any nuggets of positive news from my research I shared with her. There are plenty of nuggets around and the time taken to explore them together takes up empty space. When the shine fades from one, another presents itself for study. We now had a shared mission and goal, which both of us embraced with determination, and I reminded her of Leonard Cohen's song 'Anthem', which we heard him sing live in Dublin some years previously, and the famous line therein: 'There is a crack, a crack in everything / That's how the light gets in.'

It all came down now to the distractions. They became the alternative treatment. A number of family milestones were on the immediate horizon which, though now bittersweet, were vital for her to reach. Kathleen's determination and focus on this task were absolute. As for work, she believed that maintaining her professional schedule and activities was essential to her mental wellbeing, though she wondered about her ability to take on the onerous duties her new roles at the IHF and RCPI would involve. We mulled over the dilemma together. The illness might turn her into a physical wreck, but so might the treatment. There was no escaping some pain and suffering. The question was whether to leave the stage and take a timeout – soft language to ease the transition to a graceful but final retreat – or to stand and play the field until she dropped. We decided on the latter approach, she because of her selfless bravery and me because of my selfish fear.

Kathleen's wig acquisitions were a great boost to her and encouraged her to go for it. As her two sisters recall, she had wanted the 'hair thing' sorted just in case. They spent a long time in the wig shop to ensure she got the best match in colour, fit and style to preserve her image and looks. She managed the situation as if it was just another shopping spree. At home that evening, she asked me if I noticed anything about her.

'No, Mum, I think you are looking well.'

'Yes, but do you notice anything different?'

I was unsure where this was going. 'Like what?'

'My hair,' she said.

'It looks great.'

To which came her reply: 'It's a wig.'

'I don't believe you!' It was an unwitting response, but it worked wonders!

'It was very expensive but I will get something back from the VHI.' (This was our private medical insurance company.)

'I hope so,' I replied.

Her oncologist advised and supported her to continue her work and carry on in her new roles. This was a vote of confidence that convinced us the diagnosis had not switched her off overnight. Our discussion on whether she should give up alcohol was brief – we decided not to stop but to keep the situation under review! Over the early course of the treatment, we both resumed our normal routines. I continued my garden work and student tutorials, while Kathleen was busier than ever with meetings in the College and in the Irish Heart Foundation, along with her private medical consulting practice in Navan. She was also involved in some important medico-legal work at the time, including giving expert testimony at a Medical Council inquiry. Paperwork was not her forte and so I became her PA, which was an effort to help with her mundane secretarial work and a boost to my self-esteem. I continued in that role throughout her illness.

12

WHAT ELSE CAN I DO?

Inevitably when you are diagnosed with a cancer, all the usual questions arise. Was I in some way responsible and at fault? Were my diet and lifestyle wrong? What about all the attention that is now focused on cancer diets? It is ironic that I have long been a strong advocate of dietary changes to reduce the risk of death from cardiovascular diseases. Can I now fix my cancer problem by changing my diet?

There has been a recent proliferation of dietary advice for cancer patients, some good, some bad and some dangerous. The temptation to manipulate one's diet is at least a way to exert some influence on the progression of the disease. Some of the dietary advice is evidence based and comes from reputable sources. Much, however, comes from less reliable sources. Diets which recommend reducing carbohydrate intake and increasing fat intake have been condemned by medical and nutritional experts. The shortage of qualified oncology dietitians compounds the problem, and leaves the way open for all manner of practitioners to fill the void.

I myself became fascinated by the Chris Wark video series on YouTube. A young man who has beaten Stage 3 colon cancer, he underwent surgery but refused chemotherapy, and instead relied on 'cancer diets' and natural therapies. He commenced a diet of fruits and vegetables, and avoided all processed foods and animal products. The difficulty with these extreme diets is that they involve exclusion of essential components of most balanced diets. Dairy products are often forbidden, yet they are essential to good health and wellness, particularly in a cancer patient being treated with chemo and hormone therapy. There were times during my treatment when I became anaemic and my white cell and platelet counts dropped. I also developed osteoporotic fractures in two of my thoracic vertebrae.

I am sure dairy exclusion would have been very unwise in my case. A good, balanced diet is also important for maintaining muscle tone, and plenty of protein and exercise facilitates this. I cannot imagine how a plant-based diet would help to stave off cachexia [weight loss, muscle wasting and increasing frailty] during prolonged chemotherapy.

Cancer patients are a very susceptible and vulnerable group and, in the absence of oncology dieticians, are likely to be influenced by stories of cures achieved as a result of organic wholefood diets and alternative therapies. However, you have to be cautious in interpreting dietary and lifestyle advice from unorthodox and non-evidenced sources.

Kathleen was an accomplished dietary guru herself, and some of her own food fads did not appear in Chris Wark's lexicon. She was a fan of bulk buying, which was a singular characteristic not just confined to food items. The same happened with clothes, garden and fashion magazines, plants and flowers and, though costly, these addictions were benign and generally off-limits to me. She could eat anything, and when she went shopping she bought everything. She always got annoyed when I remarked she had brought too much food home and was never happy when I went shopping with her. I excused myself from this chore early on in our married life, but when she became ill, I felt obliged to resume it. It did not work out and I was stood down again!

When it came to food and drink, Kathleen had a number of quirky habits. She liked the taste of tea but only fully drank her morning cup. During the day she made multiple cups of tea, took one or two sips and then left near-full cups all over the house, which I collected each evening. She was a salt and vinegar woman and, rather than sprinkling salt and vinegar on any type of hot potato, she poured both onto the unsuspecting Irish vegetable and most of these additives ended up in the bin. Her benchmark for drinking wine was an abstemious surgeon classmate whom she admired, and who once told her he drank one glass of wine each evening with his dinner, which kept him in shape in mind and in body. Somehow this gave her licence to drink at will, and both of us had more than the occasional binge on weekdays and weekends (when we were off duty, of course).

Alternative therapies including cancer diets had to be considered and none could be totally discarded. We both believed finding the primary was our only realistic chance of modifying and slowing the disease's progression. Chris Wark's 'cure', and most of the cures supposedly achieved through diet and other non-conventional therapies, occurred in patients who had already had surgery and then decided to refuse chemotherapy in favour of these alternative treatments, particularly cancer diets. They were in a far better place than Kathleen because their survival odds with surgery alone were already high. We did, however, set some store by her wellbeing stats. She had a good appetite and a very stable normal weight. I had always found these markers of wellbeing very reliable in my practice, and the subsequent reassurance provided to patients allowed them to better cope with their illness and remain positive. I used to welcome news from her that she had put on weight – but my satisfaction on this score did not always please her! Many of Kathleen's close colleagues also remarked honestly on her healthy appearance, and it did provide both of us with some comfort throughout most of her illness. It also prompted me to examine her dietary habits with renewed interest.

Since my diagnosis, I have of course very kindly been offered numerous suggestions about available treatments and therapies – diet, spiritual and religious renewal, lifestyle changes, in addition to therapies available in other parts of the world. I have attempted to evaluate the evidence for each, where it exists, and how it might impact on my situation.

There is much written in the lay press about the encouraging results of some new treatments but these relate to patients with a particular kind of cancer diagnosis. In my case there is no clear management plan available for treating my cancer. Unknown to myself, I had an advanced cancer well before my diagnosis was made. When confronted with this devastating news, I ask – why me? What have I done in my lifestyle or work life that might have brought this on, with all the attendant guilt?

Coping with cancer is difficult. I am sure being a doctor patient is the worst scenario for both the treating doctor and the patient. For me, the diagnosis of an unknown cancer, or CUP, has been particularly difficult, as it does not fit with my lifelong management approach with sick patients, i.e., examine, diagnose, treat. At least there is then a road map to follow. I don't even have that to lean on. My only good fortune is that my medical 'performance status' and level of fitness has allowed me to pursue some of my professional activities and this has helped me to stay sane in the head so far.

It was now time to put both of our life's memories and experience to work, to reflect on the joys and the pains that got us here and the wisdom gained from battles won and lost. We were still focusing our efforts on trying to make the primary diagnosis, while the doctors had moved on to the stage of 'treat the patient'. We discussed our findings in bed at night, but the more research we did, the less we learned.

'We know it is going to be a rocky road, Mum, but let's go with what Des tells us.'

That was what she wanted to hear.

'OK, Dad, I agree.'

The other actor always hovering in the wings was loneliness, a constant companion of all of us, but one rarely acknowledged in the good times. Reading was a private affair, a space for personal reflection and a source of consolation for Kathleen, much as lighting candles was for me. We shared praying and gardening, but I had more time and need for these and so did more of each. These activities provided mental comfort and light relief and, when added to travel and treatment time, took up most of our waking hours.

We both knew the natural history of most of the common diseases, including the cancers, and the benefits of different interventions. In general, the more diagnostic information that is available, the better the outcome. Our dilemma was that in Kathleen's case there was less information available and, therefore, it followed that the outcome would be less favourable. We were the main actors in the play; too close to the action, we had lost the plot and were in a constant search for answers. And any answers we did receive had to be parsed. We knew that if the response to the question 'Will it work?'

is 'It's worth a try', this means it won't work! We knew that a long investigation report crammed with information often means the specialty reviewers do not know what is wrong and that the report is inconclusive.

The default position for the informed patient is to ask, 'What would you do, Doctor, if you were in my position?' The uninformed patient, on the other hand, is still inclined to say, 'I will go along with whatever you think is best, Doctor,' and even today that is often a wise choice! Kathleen was inclined to adopt that latter course because in her practice she spent so much time weighing up the management and treatment options that she was providing personalised advice and a tailored treatment plan for each patient. In this, she was ahead of her time. Today the buzzwords in cancer care are 'precision medicine' and 'targeted treatment', based on information about the behaviour of certain genes that change or mutate and misbehave in a medical world where the individual genetic make-up of the patient can be determined. Kathleen's hope was that this new dawn would come to her rescue.

Grasping at straws is a surprising pastime that gave us occasional moments of relief. 'Dad, I read an article in *Time* magazine today about a new treatment for cancer.' The frequent small advances in cancer research often get big headlines in the press. They regularly raise false hopes and mislead, but for a short time they can be manna for the mind and the soul. They are worth the few hours of exploration they prompt before the bubble bursts. Such precious interludes were for us an opportunity for a glass of wine and a smile. Don't ever tell anyone there is no hope. If you do and take away their illusion, you only compound their loneliness and they lose their will to live. After the glass of wine, we always mounted our bikes again!

13

OFF WE GO, ON A WING AND A PRAYER

I commenced the chemo on 16 May 2016. I was unable to tolerate Oxaliplatin. Four hours after the first infusion dose, I developed acute dramatic neuritis [nerve pain] – sudden acute painful burning paraesthesia [pins and needles] in my hands and feet – and next morning I could not write or even sign my name. I was not expecting this, and got quite a fright. At Finbar's request, I phoned the nurse on call and she said she would inform my oncology doctor. Neuropathy [loss of sensation, 'pins and needles' and sometimes balance] is more common but not as dramatic, but I also had long-standing restless legs which aggravated things. These symptoms continued for over a week; I also had intermittent back pain and a cough. I received an abnormal blood test report in the post which caused me more anxiety. I felt miserable.

I started on an inhaler for my cough. I watched the movie Snapshots *with Finbar one evening, and it was nice to be watching it together as Finbar was never a movie fan. My oncologist phoned me on 27 May, and told me he was going to change the chemo. He stopped the Oxaliplatin and I continued on the 5FU and Leucovorin. This combination was more tolerable, despite plenty of gastrointestinal side effects. I kept lip balm in the pocket of every coat for use between Days 4 and 7 post-chemotherapy. The magic hospital nausea medication and the Dexamethasone (a steroid) were a great help, and I determined with Finbar's help to lead as normal a life as possible.*

The Oxaliplatin episode shook our confidence and I could see Kathleen was scared of the neurological side-effects, which, if they continued, would limit her ability to carry on with any work activity. She was equally worried that by stopping the drug the chances of slowing the progression of the cancer would be diminished. The other two drugs had been standard generic cancer treatments for years. She did not have a standard cancer, however, but an aggressive one with no name, so she faced the prospect of depending on a sub-optimal combination of drugs. I spent some more time on the internet and was relieved that the evidence was strong that 5FU and Leucovorin were worthwhile and of proven benefit. This was subsequently confirmed by her oncologist when she returned for her next chemo session. The best treatment for her at the time was to become immersed in her clinical and professional work activities, and with gentle prompting, that is what she did.

Kathleen's chemotherapy cycles were initially planned for twelve weeks with treatment doses scheduled every two weeks. She had to be in the Mater Private Hospital at 7.45 a.m., and we always planned to arrive at 7.30 a.m. The rationale that the earlier you arrived, the sooner you were finished and ready to go did not always hold true, but that was our routine. It meant getting up at 5.30 a.m. and leaving no later than 6.15 a.m.

One of her lifelong benign ailments was IBS (irritable bowel syndrome), and this was aggravated by the chemotherapy. She also had a weak bladder and so we had to identify the rest stops on the way to Dublin, as the urgency to go to the loo could strike with little warning. It was fortunate that there was a 24/7 filling station with toilet facilities halfway along the route, which served us well and often. I would fill up the tank with petrol or diesel while she would buy the newspaper and a magazine and head for the bathroom. In some filling stations you had to ask for a key to access the toilet, so in such an establishment you felt obliged to buy something and become a patron!

Public toilets in Ireland are like warm, sunny spells on a rainy day – few and far between. Hotels and public houses are inundated with visitors seeking to use their facilities. Most of these are women and they are usually accommodated, though often with a visible degree of annoyance or reluctance on the part of the proprietor or manager. New hotels are responding to this nuisance by placing the toilets in more discreet areas to deter bathroom-only guests. Kathleen was always a persistent offender and in good times had delighted in sampling the facilities in top fancy hotels. I remember her visiting the Ritz and Hôtel de Crillon in Paris during a weekend trip, while I nervously window-shopped on the street outside. I was more likely to come under scrutiny than she! She was able to go from the sublime to the ridiculous, as on our annual summer holidays in Connemara, where she was often reduced to seeking relief in the long grass on the rock-face hill on Lettergesh beach or the sandy dunes in Glassilaun. On these occasions, I would be posted on sentry duty for the duration!

The second problem about our early-morning journeys to the hospital was to ensure we arrived safely, and that was a feat in itself. I was a good driver but the commuter traffic along the two-way secondary roads from our home to Dublin demanded total concentration, ingenuity and prayer to survive each morning. I always drove just inside the speed limit, but I was overtaken by every car en route and was reminded of my tardiness and of the nuisance I was causing my fellow drivers by the constant flashing of lights in my rear-view mirror. Only in Ireland could you imagine that in this mix you could be simultaneously confronted by the flashing lights of oncoming traffic warning you of Garda checkpoints on the route ahead.

During this period, we had to find something to keep us going that was reliable and could be measured. Prayers, Masses, Novenas and candles were all very well but were for further down the road – except, of course, for the candles I had been burning for quite some time already.

'What do you think, Dad?'

'You look well, you are up and about and as busy as ever,' I would reply. 'Your appetite is fine and your weight is steady. That's good enough for me.'

She could not argue with that assessment and it provided some reassurance to both of us.

For Kathleen, the other indicators she placed some stock in were the routine blood tests performed before her chemo treatments and repeated at each session. When I collected her, my first question was always, 'What's the news, Mum?' And she would say all was well, with a wan accompanying smile, and I'd squeeze her hand in grateful acknowledgement. Over the first year of treatment, her haemoglobin, platelet and white cell counts remained within the normal range on most occasions, and so her chemo went ahead as planned. We sometimes celebrated the small 'win' with a coffee in a nearby café in Dorset Street before heading home.

As her self-appointed PA, I adjusted quickly to my new role. My duties included delivering her prescriptions to the pharmacy in Navan, often returning later in the day to collect the medicine. In between, I'd cut the grass and do some weeding in the garden. I was also, of course, her 'chemo driver', and while waiting to bring her home after her treatment I would spend time in the on-campus library surfing the internet for 'the cure', and for relaxation, I conducted bedside tutorials with the hospital's medical students.

After Kathleen had recovered from the scary peripheral neuropathy symptoms, the normal pattern of debilitating chemotherapy side-effects kicked in. Her ongoing left flank and back pain and a troublesome cough were more distressing, and as a result her anxiety levels remained high. Later that month a blood test result arrived in the post out of the blue with more bad news. Her C191 marker was abnormal. Her gynaecologist, who had arranged some unrelated screening tests, had sent it on to her. While non-specific, C191 markers are often very high in patients with pancreatic cancer.

I played down the significance of this result and reassured her. Fortunately her mind was busy at the time, as she was acting as an expert witness in a Medical Council inquiry and had to write a detailed report before giving her evidence. I helped her by advising on the presentation and format and correcting her grammar! In the middle of all this turmoil, she was continuing to see some private patients in her Navan clinic. She drove to and from Navan to maintain her 'motor' autonomy and control, and would return home with a collection of flowerpots in the boot of the car for my attention. That month of May ended with a visit to her dentist and the welcome news that Ruth's 20-week scan was normal.

I met Barry Dempsey, CEO of the Irish Heart Foundation, to make arrangements for the 50 years' celebrations of the founding of the Irish Heart Foundation. I have to give a speech at the Irish President's official home, Áras an Uachtaráin, on 06/09/2016. Will I be well enough? Will all my hair be gone? Mentally, these jobs are good for me. My doctor's advice is to continue with normal life as much as possible. Can I manage life in the public eye with a wig? My hair, which was my 'crowning glory', has gone very thin. I must get photos taken for IHF magazine before it all falls out.

The early-morning drives to Dublin increased in June 2016, as the Irish Heart Foundation's board had two special meetings to coordinate its anniversary-year activities. At the same time, plans for moving to a new headquarters were gathering pace. Kathleen was also busy attending to her duties in the RCPI. However, fatigue and mouth ulcers and loose teeth were taking a toll on her health. A new complaint of an exquisitely tender finger forced her on one occasion to attend the emergency department in Navan. The X-ray was normal.

Kathleen's father's health deteriorated steadily during this time but she visited him as often as she could; after dropping her to his home in Mount Merrion, I usually walked up to the local church to pray and light candles. On the last weekend in June, when we were away down the country, Grandad McGarry took a turn for the worse. We returned to Dublin and fortunately Kathleen was able to be with him the evening before he died.

14

GRANDAD GONE

In the middle of this, Grandad died. The eulogy our nephew John read at the funeral accurately described the great man he was. Grandad had recurrent chest infections and each time he was treated with antibiotics he developed C. Diff. diarrhoea, which was a dreadful affliction. He had recently been hospitalised and it caused me great heartache that I was unable to visit him as often as I wished, because of my increased susceptibility to infections due to my chemo treatment. It was a relief for all the family that he died peacefully at home surrounded by his loved ones.

He was fortunate that he had a state pension and some savings that allowed him to fund his own care, with some home care assistance from the HSE. His funeral was a joyful event and all the grandchildren took part in the ceremonies. He was buried in Burren cemetery in Warrenpoint beside my mother, Kathleen, who died in 2014, and her infant brother, John. Another of my mother's brothers, Professor Denis Donoghue, a well-known academic, has written a memoir of his childhood in Warrenpoint.

I had one of my chemo treatments the day before the funeral, but it was a good day for me as I get a dose of steroids for two days, which gives me a boost before the side effects commence. It is a great change to lose the second parent. The family home is no longer a focus to meet. Even in later years I still remember asking Grandad, as we called him, for advice and direction as he was such a wise and kind man. I am glad he never knew about my diagnosis of cancer. We told him I had some stomach troubles and he puzzled over that. I am so relieved neither of my parents knew what became of me, as they would have been devastated.

My own family was so blessed that both my parents lived to be over 90, in relatively good health, and successfully as a team completing the Irish Times *crossword virtually until the day they died. This good fortune is related to genes, good medical care and sufficient resources to provide care in the home. Not all are so lucky and the spectacle of the elderly lying on trolleys in EDs, awaiting admission, continues for so many and is totally unacceptable. Many have illnesses that could be treated with antibiotics at home if adequate resources were provided to the country's Primary Care Service.*

Grandad was 91 when he died; 'Granny Garry' had been 92. When they reach that age, they pass away. It is only the young that could be said to die. They are wrenched away, with gloom and sadness, whereas the leaving of those who live well into old age is celebrated with joy and tears of gratitude. Grandad and Granny were happy for one more day!

Just before Grandad's 90th birthday, I penned this poem for him, written from the perspective of Granny Garry – who was one year his senior:

I remember yesterday.
It was cold and I stayed indoors
on my kitchen chair.
Kevin is always with me.
I know because he never stops talking.
He still remembers 60 years ago,
Probably more, but 60 is enough.
I know he has always been jealous of my age.
He married an older woman
at a time when that was frowned upon.
I look forward to celebrating
his coming-of-age at 90,
when we will be the same.

Granny and Grandad already knew all about Kathleen and what she meant to them. They were hugely proud of her. She had excelled in everything she did from the day she was born and looked after both of them until the day they died. They knew she had reached all the important milestones in life and were there with her to celebrate each of them. They also knew that everybody is going to die sometime, and kept the faith – and so did she. Shortly after Grandad died, Kathleen attended the funeral of Professor Risteárd Mulcahy, one of the founders and the first President of the IHF, who was one of her teachers and mentors. She joined the congregation in celebrating his professional and academic milestones and then with renewed energy got on with her own life again.

15

THE BATTLE RAGES ON

July 2016

After five sessions of chemo, the side effects' symptoms are lasting longer. Nausea a constant after two weeks. Hair thinned and one of my teeth broke. I have had a lot of dental problems while on chemo, including a dental abscess, a subsequent molar extraction followed by a dry socket and later bits of teeth and then whole teeth falling out. Horrors – will all my teeth fall out? My wonderful dentist in Navan saw me again at a moment's notice and managed to cobble together a temporary replacement. Hopefully there will be chance to fix eventually. I spent as much time in the dentist's chair as I did on the chemo ward! All these things have been a major strain on me – sans hair, sans teeth, sans everything. Whether I am going to the grave or not, I am not going there without my front teeth.

'Is the treatment working?' 'Am I getting better?' 'Is the cancer under control?' These were questions that were constantly on her mind, but which she never asked out loud. Instead, she framed her questions in a different way. 'Will I see my first grandchild?' 'Will I be well enough to attend the marriage of my son David?' 'Will I see my second grandchild?' These milestone events took place as her illness progressed, and indeed her oncologist took his cue from her and was more comfortable relating to her in this nuanced language – something which I thought worked well at the time. He modified the treatment schedule to accommodate her and ensure as best he could that she would be fit enough to enjoy each of them. Meanwhile, I was doing my best to manage her diet, and my new smoothie creations were well received and literally swallowed whole. Her appetite remained good and her weight steady, as they say in the vernacular. But none of this could disguise the fact that the disease was winning, and both of us could read between the lines. Though we did not admit to it and clung to the belief that we had to be patient to experience the benefits of chemo, her decline had commenced.

Our downtime and most of our happy hours were spent in the garden, our place of sanctuary and haven of hope. There the plants and flowers vied with the restful open spaces of green, well-trimmed plots, as the old tall trees drooped and bent their heavy branches low around us. Kathleen never saw the weeds, nor did she seem interested in them. At one point I decided to put my head above the parapet.

'But the weeds spoil the appearance, Mum, and you know they will be the first thing John Bentley will see when you invite him up.'

'Well, why don't you get rid of them – and mind you keep away from the flowers,' she replied tartly, but with an accompanying loving smile.

Our gardener, Michael Englishby, arrived up shortly after that exchange of sweet nothings. He had come as usual to do the first 'heavy-lifting' garden work of the year. He is a hard worker and always does a good job. Kathleen would spend time with him on each visit, going through the minutiae of the garden chores just as she had done with Paddy Ward for 25 years. Michael took everything she said on board and delivered a 'Chelsea garden' to her a week later, which she loved to show off to her friends.

As part of his duties, Michael would also duplicate some of my work at times, particularly in relation to the weeds. Kathleen had never been impressed with my ability to rid the gravel pathways of the weeds, as they frequently sprouted up soon after my surgery. I knew this was par for the course but believed that constant plucking was the only way to keep weeds in check, and I did not think Michael's approach was any better. But I was not the one in charge, of course, and so she told him to just do his usual job and I decided to let him get on with it.

On the first day of Michael's efforts with the weeds, I went up to see him before he finished, to acknowledge his work. I had resisted indulging in my pastime for a few weeks so he could see the extent of the weed problem.

'You know, Michael, we never seem to be able to get on top of this problem … After about six weeks they are back in abundance.' I then told him that his last attempt, involving the immersion of the soil with the weed killer, had failed.

'That was due to the rain,' he said.

I did not press the point after this, but asked him to come back in about a month to review. There was very little rain in the interim and when he returned, without any prompting, he exclaimed surprise that the new growth was more noticeable.

'It must be they are just not making the weed killer like before,' he said.

'Yes, it's like the rinse aid for the dishwasher: it's become too dilute and too cheap,' I replied. I thought we were finally on the same wavelength, until his next statement.

'You shouldn't have started pulling them again for ten days to allow the weed killer to work on them.'

He might have been right, and perhaps his neo-adjuvant treatment had been foiled by hasty surgical intervention!

❖

The course of Ruth's pregnancy remained stable, and she came home frequently to be with Mum and to spend her money in Mothercare on all the necessities for a new baby. Meanwhile, I spent my money on candles in any church I found on my travels. In mid-July we set off for our annual holiday to Connemara. Kathleen got sick on the way down and had to spend a day in bed. We returned home because her pain and nausea was getting worse. We got a boost, however, a few days later when our second son, Peter, announced his engagement to his girlfriend Nerea, and the news seemed to settle her symptoms for a while. On our return to Connemara one of Kathleen's teeth fell out in a restaurant, and another damper descended on us. We went home to visit the dentist and she had her review CT scan about the same time. We eventually got a break from the side-effects and she enjoyed the August bank-holiday weekend in the west without any further complications. On our return home, however, we got bad news: the CT scan results revealed that the cancer had progressed.

9 August 2016

Disaster day. CT: no improvement after first-line chemo; nodes increased in size? New node in lung. Plan to change treatment. Called Finbar and he went to discuss with DC. Disaster! Finbar emotional – me numb. Will I see my grandchild and my two sons' weddings? Hard to accept this.

Back on Thursday 11 August to start new drugs with better pancreas effect! Nurses extremely efficient, professional and careful. Plan to continue my life and fulfil my commitments.

Comment: no effect from chemo so far. Now for two new

drugs. Maybe they won't work either, and mortality? Ruth's baby in 8 weeks. Don't want to worry her. Latest concern: herpes can be transmitted to newborns (Irish Times). More anxiety.

How to cope?

1. *Finbar brilliant and supportive.*
2. *Organise my home and jewellery, in case of worst. Label jewellery for brides in 2017. Jewellery for Ruth (baby). Fix my engagement ring. Things to do and organise: I have been organising all my life and this will help me.*
3. *At least I feel the kids are on the road to being sorted out now. Stable relationships and jobs and my parents both at rest.*

In April when I got my diagnosis, I wondered if I would see my grandchild. There is no relief from cancer. Some people say there can be positives – appreciating little things more and appreciating nature and loved ones. I am sure this is true, but I am not seeing it this year. I want to be well for my daughter's first baby (my first grandchild) on 4/10/2016. It is a high-risk pregnancy as she has thrombophilia [abnormal clotting of the blood] and is on Clexane [an anticoagulant drug prescribed in pregnancy].

Kathleen started her new chemo regime on 11 August. I spoke to Des Carney, the oncologist. We were more than colleagues but less than close friends. We had known each other for a long time and got on well, and so it could be said that we were 'medical friends'. I understood and could parse his language, which wisely left a lot of burning questions unanswered. I also knew from my early consultant days that doctors are not infallible – apart from my late surgical mentor, of course, who, after acknowledging that fact in the declarative sentence, would invariably conclude with the phrase 'But I am never wrong'!

Following my conversation with DC, I realised that things had not really changed and the battle raged on for both of us. There were moments when our resolve faltered, but only moments. While the new chemo was being poured into Kathleen's body, I was in a jewellery shop on Grafton Street, buying her an eternity ring.

I have just started the new chemo regime – Gemzar. What if I don't tolerate it: what then? Anxious times. It's better not to know every side effect. The nurse told me it's very unlikely I will get a neuropathy.

I have a very busy schedule in the IHF, RCPI and in the private rooms. How will I manage? Finbar is very good and is doing most of the driving, though I still want to be able to drive to Navan, to attend the rooms, to shop and to go to see my wonderful dentist and pharmacist.

I have mixed feelings about religion but I have promised to visit Sr Briege Mc Kenna, the healing nun, the next time she is in Ireland.

Some of the side-effects of the chemo on this occasion were new, including diarrhoea, acid reflux, sore lips and occasional chest pain, and so we had something different to search for on the internet and discuss in bed at night. During this brief period of introspection, I was called back to the future to attend another surgical emergency. This time, the phone call in the middle of the night was successfully transmitted to the new bedroom extension. It was from May, Paddy's wife, to summon me to their home in the village where Paddy had suddenly taken ill. Paddy was then 101 and had never spent a night in hospital. Even though he was in extreme distress, he intended to hold on to this record with his life! In the end, however, after we had browbeaten him into submission, he finally agreed and I arranged an ambulance to bring him into the local hospital.

August was a busy month, and towards its end, Kathleen met a 'healing nun' in All Hallows, Dublin's famous seminary. The following day, after escorting her into another chemo session, I came out to find my car clamped. I went over to Berkeley Road Church to light some candles, but they did not work and I had to pay the 80 euro fine!

In the early days of September, we worked together on her IHF speeches, between more visits to the dentist, and then made another trip to keep Ruth company in Edinburgh (where she now lived) for a few late-pregnancy days. At the end of that month, Professor Frank Murray, the RCPI president, warmly thanked Kathleen for her 25 years of service to the College at a special meeting for the occasion, which was followed shortly by another party held in her honour at Collon House. There was much reminiscing there about days of yore, when her hilarious and hysterical fits of laughter would herald random joyful moments in her life — for example, during my recitation of poems that I had composed on paper napkins between courses at dinner parties. Our wedding anniversary celebrations on 1 October were low-key that year, as we headed off to Edinburgh to welcome our first grandchild into the world.

16

FINN ARRIVES AND WINTER COMES AGAIN

Finbar and I arranged to stay in an Airbnb traditional Edinburgh flat, and were there when Finn was born in the Edinburgh Royal Infirmary. He was a most beautiful baby with an Apgar score of 9/10 [a test for newborns based on five key criteria for wellness], and it was great to see him at only a few hours old. We celebrated together that evening in the Balmoral Hotel in Princes Street. It was a lovely exciting time and I was grateful to be there.

Ruth's baby was due on 4 October 2016. We arrived in Edinburgh on 30 September to a very nice Airbnb apartment, but it was on the top floor with a stone staircase and no lift. We were both short of breath after the climb, but Kathleen noticeably more so. 'Phew, that was hard work,' she said. I feigned equal distress and promised next time to make sure we paced ourselves and took a short breather halfway up. Later that day, a visit to the zoo presented a similar problem, which we solved by taking the bus to the summit and doing the tour back to front – or, more aptly, top to bottom.

Ruth was admitted to the Royal Infirmary on the morning of 5 October, after her waters broke. Her anticoagulants were stopped so she could have an epidural. There was little advance in her labour during the course of the day, and when we visited that evening, she told us the plan was to wait another 12 hours before any active intervention was contemplated. We were anxious about the delay but returned to the apartment and went to bed. We received a call from Ruth's husband, Paddy, sometime after 7 a.m. the next morning to tell us that she had delivered a baby boy.

Mum's delight and relief were a joy to behold. I hugged her tightly and felt her pent-up tension drain away. It was a moment of spinning change for both of us, perhaps something like a spiritual essence. Kathleen's happiness was always expressed effusively, with loud exclamations and gestures of acclaim, in contrast to my typically underwhelming way of acknowledging joy or contentment, with measured tones and smiles.

'It's fantastic news, Finbar – it's our first grandchild! Let's go and see him!'

'Well, let's get ready first, Mum, and have breakfast.'

It was a totally inadequate response to her clarion call, but she knew she was dealing with the man who had an unusual track record in dealing with first-born infants and wanted to ensure there was no slip-up on his part this time. In any case, after breakfast we caught the bus to the hospital as planned and were able to meet our beautiful first grandchild later that morning. When we arrived on the hospital ward, all seemed calm and well. He looked great and we each got to hold him.

Nothing was ever plain sailing with Ruth. She recounted the events of the previous 12 hours to Mum, whose joy was now mixed with consternation. As I have mentioned, Ruth was on subcutaneous anticoagulation medication throughout her pregnancy, which she self-injected twice daily; because she wanted to have the option of an epidural, her anticoagulants had been discontinued the previous evening. Her pre-delivery monitoring included ultrasound imaging of the baby *in utero*, and during the night the cord was noted floating about the baby's neck, and he was having short bouts of foetal distress. And so Ruth was prepped in case she needed an emergency caesarean section. Instead, she had a difficult forceps delivery, which was successful.

Kathleen's clinical antennae over the following 48 hours forewarned that Ruth might have developed a pulmonary embolus (a clot in the lungs), as her pulse rate was very high and none of the usual post-partum causes of a tachycardia were evident. At the time of her forceps delivery, she had been off her anticoagulant medication for a full 24 hours, and Kathleen surmised that this procedure might have disturbed Ruth's pelvic venous system and released a small clot from the site of her pelvic DVT from ten years earlier. After delivery, she had been put back on a reduced dose of anticoagulants, but Kathleen's concern was that this was insufficient at this stage if there was indeed a clot forming. We knew that consultants try to steer clear of relatives, particularly in the hospital setting, but Kathleen found a discreet legitimate communication route to ensure that her suspicion was passed on to the haematology team for consideration – and a significant increase in the dose of anticoagulants soon followed. They made this decision based on the clinical findings without performing a confirmatory CT pulmonary scan, in the knowledge she would resume her ante-partum dosage in any event. In the circumstances, this was a wise and sensible decision and reduced Ruth's well-concealed anxiety and her parents' overt concern. It confirmed in Kathleen's mind that her daughter was in good and expert hands.

Ruth's doctors told her she probably did have a small pulmonary embolus post-partum, but she got over it and they have decided to continue her anticoagulation medication as before and not do any more tests. I am glad and relieved for Ruth and Paddy. They must have been worried but did not show it.

Kathleen was truly a 'world authority' on coagulation disorders and their treatment, ever since Ruth's life-threatening major pelvic DVT a decade previously. She had studied the literature on every aspect of the condition and attended at least one major international conference each year. Following Ruth's illness, we had discovered that our family was populated with carriers of the Factor 5 Leiden Deficiency gene. Kathleen was into genes and, in fact, had been a principal participating member of an international team that had been able to identify a unique gene in a large Irish family with hypertrophic cardiomyopathy. She had treated many members of this family in the cardiology department of Our Lady's Hospital, Navan.

In any case, crisis averted, we stayed on in Edinburgh until Ruth's pulse rate settled and she was feeling a good deal better. We saw more of the baby and took pictures on our phones to confirm that all was real and we had become proud grandparents at last.

We made another visit to Edinburgh to see Ruth, Finn and Paddy in early November. On our return home, Kathleen began fretting about her next scan, due on the 14th. Given her recent preoccupation with Ruth's post-partum problems, perhaps she now had scans on the brain! With no news still three days after her scan, she sent a text to her doctor.

'He probably does not know the result himself, Mum. The Mater is a different set-up to what you had in Navan. I am sure he will get back to you very soon.'

He texted her to say he would call her the next day.

'Does he not know how worried I am? It must be bad news,' she said.

'I am sure he is off to discuss it with the radiologist,' I replied and gave her a hug.

We stopped at our usual filling station the following morning on our way to Dublin. As I waited for her in the car outside, she came out of the shop to tell me that her consultant had phoned to say there had been no further progression. She was relieved and smiling. I drove her to the RCPI for her meeting, and we went out to a local restaurant that evening to 'celebrate'!

Waiting for news was a source of stress for both of us. For Kathleen, the anxiety commenced at the time of, and during the course of, the test. The phlebotomist generally took more blood than she expected because there were more bottles to fill. The radiographer took extra views of her chest and abdomen and, when asked to explain, would often say it was because she did not stay still in the CT chamber. Occasionally, when she unwisely asked her about the size of the glands, she would sometimes reply, 'I got them,' whatever that meant. Reassurance was in short supply, but of course it was unrealistic to expect it from phlebotomists or radiographers.

Kathleen found it difficult to have to wait so long at times for news of her test results, as a doctor herself, who had spent so much of her life explaining in real time to patients and their relatives what was wrong. For her, the longer the wait, the more likely that the news was bad. In the case of a doctor-patient like Kathleen, perhaps a short time lapse was understandable, as the results were likely first discussed with a number of the primary consultant's colleagues before she would receive the definitive word. The effect of the delay on her was always traumatic – as it was on me, but my job was to try and explain the delay, and reassure her.

I have sympathy in these situations for the primary consultant, who is in a difficult place, as the patient's expectation is that once the test is done the result should be available shortly thereafter. It does not work like that anymore. During my own time in practice, I recall beating a path mid-afternoon to the radiology and pathology departments and knocking on colleagues' doors looking for that morning's results. They were always helpful but I am sure, with hindsight, they felt intimidated, particularly when dealing with an impatient, short-fused colleague, often a surgeon like me, expecting instant answers. The introduction of multidisciplinary meetings has changed all that. Definitive results and management plans are not finalised until each case is discussed and the findings and treatment are agreed by all. Such cross-specialty discussions facilitate a greater sense of combined objective care and also tend to reduce the inflated egos of some impatient surgeons. This process however inevitably leads to delays for the unfortunate patient, but generally ensures that reliable, evidence-based decisions are made.

2016 drew to a close with Finn's christening in Kilkenny, followed by the usual full programme of the Lennon and McGarry families' traditional Christmas celebrations in Collon.

Kathleen increased her analgesic intake to keep her pain-free for the duration. It was another milestone reached and passed. She asked me to bring her to the post-Christmas Arnotts sale in Dublin to indulge in her favourite pastime. I benefited too because she bought me a new suit, two pairs of trousers and two ties. She also bought another new outfit for herself to be stored in one of her many wardrobes for future use!

17

JOY AND SUFFERING

I want to be well for my son David's wedding to Caroline in May 2017. I want to have more time with my darling husband Finbar, who has been so unbelievably supportive – our combined sense of humour has been a great help as well as his determination to keep me positive. These are targets, but will I make them?

To have cancer as a doctor is a double whammy, as every ache and pain is magnified in the mind and becomes cancer cells whizzing around the body. I have avoided the internet and decided to do what the doctor tells me. Finbar has taken to the internet but no really good news. We have read all the dietary/mindfulness/holy books. I have embarked on a healthier diet – smoothies, vegetables and so on. I have not embraced 'special' diets because at the moment I am concerned with maintaining my weight to endure the chemo. There are many reports of individual remissions

apparently relating to diet but with my training in Clinical
Pharmacology, I have to be sceptical when the numbers do
not add up.

The early months of 2017 were difficult for Kathleen, not just because of the physical toll of the chemotherapy but also because of the mental distress as to why she was still being given it. Back pain, fatigue, persistent pain in her arm at a vaccination site and ongoing nausea featured frequently in my diary entries in January and February (I kept a journal too at the time, with brief notes pertaining to Kathleen's illness).

'Dad, maybe we should be thinking about immunotherapy?' With this, I knew she had begun to browse the internet without permission.

'Are you losing faith in my smoothies, and Sue, John, Aileen and Irene's meals-on-wheels, not to mention Rosemary's Masses and Novenas?'

Trump's inauguration events on TV provided a new distraction. Social pageants and public occasions were a lifelong fascination for Kathleen, and these celebrations were a change from her normal preoccupation with the British royal family. Her mood plummeted again at the end of January, after listening to extensive media coverage on pancreatic cancer. 'That's what I have, Dad,' she said sadly. I learned that responses don't always have to be vocal and sometimes an equivocal nod or smile can convey reassurance. There is some merit in the emojis, after all.

When Kathleen's dear friend Arthur died of cancer a week later, she was very upset. He had taken an interest in the schoolboy rugby careers of our three boys, and in return during the time of his illness, I had often lit candles for him in Berkeley Road Church, for which he was grateful. Along with him and his wife Anne, we were part of a surgical group called the Club of 13. It had 26 members, as all the spouses were 'paid-up' members and full participants in its activities. A few of us were outliers or 'country cousins', including my good friend Bosco, who had also died from cancer, but the mix of talents worked very well. The accomplished metropolitan surgeons, many of whom were professors, were always somewhat diffident in reminding us of their status and titles. The resultant dynamic offered opportunities for fun and banter. I am reminded of what an old wily Franciscan said many moons ago: 'My dear Finbar, I may not have gone to school but I met the scholars coming home.'

By way of contrast, Kathleen was a member of another medical club called the Eclectic Physicians, who were distinguished from their surgical colleagues by their perceived cognitive abilities and relative humility. Only in retirement did they finally achieve the work–life balance that had eluded them when they needed it most. The majority, like Kathleen, had worked on busy rotas in small and medium-sized hospitals outside Dublin. Not surprisingly, only one or two of them were professors, but in their bases in the towns and regions they were well regarded and respected , and were all hailed as 'professors' within the community.

❖

Fundraising was an important part of Kathleen's new role in the Irish Heart Foundation, and in early 2017 she hosted the inaugural regional charity lunch in Navan, surrounded by many grateful patients and their families as well as corporate supporters from the town and locality. She spoke about the risk factors associated with heart disease and stroke. Her speech was crafted to send subliminal, sage advice to young men and women, including her own children and sibs, who were present for the occasion. She and I never smoked but our three boys did and were slow to acknowledge the expert advice on their doorstep.

When it came to health matters, Kathleen was a champion of prevention, and quitting smoking is a no-brainer if you want to reduce your risk of premature death from heart disease and cancer. Smart guys don't smoke anymore and prevention is the only cure that works – this was her constant refrain. It is unfortunate that children and young adults these days continue to smoke. It seems that Kathleen's message on smoking is not trending anymore, and the means of communicating it has to change. Maybe all that is required is the creation of a new, reformed Marlboro Man – one who frowns on smoking – to convert the target audience.

In this and so many other matters, Kathleen was a role model for our children, and she believed it was up to them to take the advice and lessons on board. She worried quietly about them but realised she could do no more and trusted they would respond. Perhaps my poem, penned in Paris in 2011 during the European Society of Cardiology Congress, which we attended together, would have a better chance of making an impression:

Salem and Winston are the incense of children.
The only visible vice observed
At the boulevard café near the Pont de Neuilly
As boys and girls gather to converse, laugh and smoke
Late afternoon in August.
Two pretty girls alone beside me
Oblivious to the old man, lean in to savour.
The cigarettes quietly stubbed out
On the legs of wooden tables
And disposed of without notice.
How long will it take
Before the warning on the packet
Leaps out and consumes them?

When we were growing up in the 1960s, old age commenced at 65 and you could count your blessings if you reached that milestone. Today, those of us who have reached 70 have been spared the ravages of premature disease. And so, by this stage we should know how to stay healthy and no longer be in need of continuing medical education. So we are now on our own in this respect and can sigh with relief. The problem these days is the sophisticated, intelligent and technologically wired people in their 30s, 40s and 50s who won't listen to or take advice. Lack of insight is a deadly malady and is difficult to cure.

❖

It was important now to establish a daily routine to help both of us cope with the dark days ahead. After the children had flown, we lived on our own in the house for ten years and spent most of the time in the kitchen, living room and two bedrooms. When Kathleen became ill, we were sleeping in separate bedrooms. It was something we had drifted into in earlier days, when I was on call and often had frequent hospital issues to deal with during the night. It allowed the other spouse to get some unbroken sleep without the interruptions of a ringing phone and whispered consultations with colleagues in the early hours of the morning. Kathleen warmed to the idea after reading books on the royal family – she noted this arrangement was commonplace and surmised if it was good enough for the Queen and Prince Philip, it was good enough for Mister and Missus Lennon! Besides which, once there were just the two of us in Greenlawns, it made sense that we should make the most of the space and each have our own room (and in Kathleen's case, dressing rooms!).

Her evening routine never changed. After looking at the TV news with me at 9 p.m., she would take a bath. We both went to bed around 10 p.m., unless there was a good film or an interesting news programme on TV, in which case she would stay up watching it. I was not a TV addict and would head upstairs after taking my pills. I would start the night off in her bed. After she took her bath and her blood-thinning injection, she would get into bed beside me and switch on her bedside light. She was a nocturnal reader and often read until 2 or 3 a.m. Her sister Pat, who was a few years younger, told me Kathleen had always been a great reader and as a child read under the bed covers with the aid of a torch after lights out.

When she was ready for sleep, she first swallowed a combination of pills including her sleeping tablets. Then she would turn to me and remark, 'It's time to repair,' which was code for me to move to my own room. I used to be a good sleeper but lost the habit when I retired. I would check back later to see if her light was still on. If she was asleep, I removed her specs, left the Kindle in her lap and turned off the light. This 'night duty' became routine during her illness. I was an early riser, and before going downstairs to prepare breakfast, I'd check on her again. On most occasions she appeared asleep and restful. In retrospect, it was the only time of the day during her illness that she was in any comfort. I had my breakfast in the kitchen and then brought her toast and tea. It was a good morning when she asked for more.

I always heard the traffic passing by early each weekday morning. This was wake-up time on chemo days and on IHF committee- and board-meeting days. I did not have an alarm clock or a watch and used to finger scroll 5 a.m. across my forehead after turning off my bedside light. It worked because I was a light sleeper and the sound of traffic signalled the arrival of morning. An occasional convoy of three or four cars could be heard passing from 5.30 a.m., and short bursts of noise would follow, with ever-diminishing silent gaps as the clock moved on. When I went to Kathleen's room to call her, she would already be up. The house was cold in the morning and she felt it more. The electric blanket kept her warm in bed, but while there were multiple sources of heat in the house, they served no useful purpose because of the draughts coming through the old windows and doors of the original house (which, as a protected property, we haven't been allowed to upgrade in any substantial way). The sooner we got out of the house, the better, as it was often warmer outside, and she got some relief from the sleep deprivation by dozing in the car.

The months between Finn's birth and David's wedding were very traumatic for Kathleen, but very busy too. Surprisingly, the coping strategy we mapped out at the outset worked well and her work with the Heart Foundation and her College was productive. She managed to discharge all her clinical and professional duties without interruption, even though she lost teeth – which each time were promptly replaced to ensure she could continue to smile at meetings with colleagues and patients. She did not miss any of her chemo sessions nor escape any of the usual side-effects, but she pre-empted the more severe and troublesome symptoms by the judicious use of additional medication, often self-prescribed. Her back pain continued to bother her but my placebo application of Difene gel at bedtime did have some beneficial effects on her mood, if not her pain. Fatigue became an issue and was managed by afternoon naps. The regular review CT scans were a constant source of anxiety for both of us. No dramatic changes were noted and the gentle nuanced information we received was that the disease's progression had slowed. This was worth the candle – and the candles – and we were happy to take our chances until the next scan arrived with further nuances to be interpreted.

18

THE NEXT LIFE

Bad Diagnosis – time to begin thinking of the next life. Religion – I do believe in the hereafter. Will I meet Granny and Grandad, Dr Sothy and Eilish O'Brien?

There were many occasions when Kathleen began conversations about 'what comes next'. They were often framed in a medical context, in terms of prognosis and the natural course of advanced disease. Patients and friends who had recently died – such as Eilish O'Brien, a community health doctor colleague of hers – were the usual prompts that she used to raise the subject. It was her way of passing on to me a message to prepare. I resisted the temptation to engage, apart from nodding and smiling to convey I understood. She seemed happy with that implied acknowledgement. She did begin to write down and itemise in detail her wishes to be discharged when the time came, who gets her jewellery, her clothes, her money. Her increasing reflective focus on her own mortality did lead me to re-examine my own faith and to seek ways of making sense of it all.

I had been writing poems all my life, some dark, some light, and now that death and the next life had moved a step closer, I sought some consolation to share with Kathleen. It's funny how the dark poems written before her illness reflected a growing sense of disenchantment, disbelief and doubt about religion. Taken together, they can be seen to be a generic commentary on a faith that for a time had lost its way. I was seeking to challenge the basic tenets of the religion I had grown up with by using contorted language for effect, for example in lines such as these: 'Eternal existence is not all it's "cracked up" to be. / Tomorrow never comes – it's always just today. / There is no night or day, just the ever now. / No name or passport, clock or compass here, / or light or beacon. / Past memories gone and all prospects blank and empty.' After illness struck and I realised the medicine was not going to work, I had to return to my roots and a new dawning and I embraced my faith again with open arms!

It is not the body that matters.
It fades and withers at the end,
a discarded badge to leave on earth.
The Soul is the character that wore it.
It will live on forever and float in the wind.

It will call by from time to time,
and watch him praying at the side altars,
burning candles for more intentions.
It will smile to acknowledge his emotions,
hoping the extra flame will buy him comfort.
'Old companion, it is fine to cry without shame.
I have not gone from you as long as you remember me.'
The goodness and kindness of that Soul
did not have to wait until she had gone.
Death does not take everything with it.

Most of our earthly rest takes place in bed. How well does it measure up to that provided in the grave? Well, at least in the grave you don't have to get up at night to turn off the light. You are no longer constantly restless because of shortness of breath. The phone does not ring to tell you a patient needs an immediate pacemaker. You don't wake up after winning the Lotto and suddenly realise it's only a dream. It is better than that because you don't wake up at all. The permutations are almost endless.

Heaven is becoming a more and more difficult eternal resting place to imagine, believe in and accept for many Catholics, as their faith has been undermined by the recent scandals in the Church. And yet it is a safe haven or refuge we desperately need when we are forced to confront our own mortality. Heaven, of course, is not a conventional place or a destination that we can understand during our short earthly existence. I wonder, for those who still believe in Heaven, whether it is manifest simply through mental gymnastics or in a form of trance; or is it only realised in the mind's eye through constant prayer and devotion to God? Is it possible to set aside sufficient dedicated time in this life for these holy pursuits to ensure we reach its portal? How to separate the angels from the fairies?

The secular, non-religious man might contemplate death and the hereafter in a very different way. Many of the memoirs I have read on death in the family and the resultant grief are written by non-believers, who are often men. The sad and traumatic experience of loss and grief forces the survivors to question the meaning of faith and religious beliefs. The eternal question is focused on whether indeed God exists. C.S. Lewis and Julian Barnes both address this question in a stark and painful way, yet bring a remorseless clarity to their analysis that, over time, is therapeutic and a source of some comfort. For them, whether or not God exists is a binary question – there are only two answers, and they are mutually exclusive. They are prepared to consider the merits of the case presented by the faithful believer and are willing to be convinced if the case is sufficiently strong. It can, however, never meet a scientific threshold and thus the answer will inevitably remain elusive, as belief and certainty are poles apart and on different circuits. This is not surprising, as mystery is a fundamental element of faith and its acknowledgement is necessary to practise as a Christian and to ensure religions survive the ages. The business of science has always been to remove the mystery. When science and rationalism square up to mystery and symbolism, they are worlds apart but are not, I believe, mutually exclusive. The former two thrive and do battle only in the earthly world we live in, whereas the latter two straddle the divide between life and death and usher in the hereafter. As long as scientists cannot fully unlock the human mind, the philosophers and poets will remain in the ascendancy – and so God has a chance.

What does the term 'a peaceful death' mean? Is it some form of supernatural state of being or existence, or an uncanny form of acute awareness that occurs as one approaches death and thus allows a prescient sense of Heaven that comforts and cradles one in that final hour? Are those who die in that state 'saved'? Are those who die with pure souls, untainted by worldly ways and who carry no burden, having fully confessed their wrongdoings, along with the children and the innocents, also safe and secure? I believe they comprise the foot soldiers or followers with 'blind faith', who have prepared for the hereafter throughout their earthly lives and accept death without any fear.

It is the essential mystery that gives 'blind faith' its currency. I believe that for practising Catholics, it is not a misnomer but an acknowledgement of their belief in God and the hereafter. Those unable to reflect on their impending death or who are so prevented by the nature of their demise, but who have lived a good life, are surely also safe and secure. True repentance if exercised by the remainder will also assure safe passage. The border crossing is between life and eternity. What comes after you cross is a mystery and, for me, is not truly relevant to the passage thereto, as your faith and hope are consumed in getting you to the border in God's grace. Once reached, you present your final mortal offering of homecoming to your Creator.

Is that not the beginning and the end of it? If you know you are heading in that direction and have the insight to understand, there is time for acknowledgement, resignation and acceptance. Those with a terminal illness can prepare and place themselves at the mercy of their God and he will answer. Does that belated preparation lead to a happy, peaceful death? If so, is that not the ultimate objective of life on earth and consistent with the prescriptive steps set out in the Bible?

If death is to have any consolation and lesson for the dying and those left behind, some of the mystery of God's plan for the faithful needs, I feel, to be delivered with more clarity and reassurance. Those who preach the Gospel have to try and convince and reassure the 'faithful' about the meaning of life and death and do so without a prepared script. Invocations of sin, suffering, fear and punishment do not work anymore. Compassion, understanding and gentle guidance and persuasion must be utilised to teach and guide the faithful along the road to redemption. That is best delivered by example. Faith is now more what you see than what you hear. It is the eyes that matter and not the words.

When Kathleen first realised what the cancer diagnosis meant for her, she remarked, 'Why me?' and after a short reflection followed with, 'Why not me?' The first is a temporal question, the second a spiritual one. We could not answer either, but it was the second question that demanded our attention. In different ways it brought our dormant faith back into relief again. We had to relearn the long-forgotten words and the songs, 'Most Sacred Heart of Jesus', 'O Immaculate Heart of Mary' and 'Ave Maria'. Though we were regular Sunday Mass goers, that was not enough to protect us from the medical condition that is most often associated with death. We did not change our overt religious routines but tried with some success to keep death at bay until we had found sufficient meaning and consolation in our Catholic religion.

19

THE CALM BEFORE THE STORM

The next joyous occasion was the wedding of my eldest son David to Caroline. They had planned the wedding for May 2017. I was not sure I would make it and I suggested bringing it forward – but they did not think that was a good idea as the plans were already in place. In early January 2017, however, David came to see me and told me they had decided after all to bring the date forward, not because of my deteriorating health but because Caroline was pregnant and was expecting a baby in July. The wedding took place in March at Richard Corrigan's gourmet paradise country estate, Virginia Park Lodge in County Cavan, and I was there with three hairpieces looking like a duchess. It was a wonderful day and I felt just like any other proud mum without a care in the world.

The 'wedding high' lasted three weeks. The weather was good and we spent a lot of time together in the garden. The children came and went and our grandson, Finn, was a special visitor who got plenty of attention. Kathleen had a lot of meetings to attend and was busy and happy. Even the review CT report did not faze her. As far as we could determine, the disease had not progressed and she decided not to ask too many questions for fear of learning more. The chemo sessions continued, as did the pain, nausea and fatigue, but she accepted this as a routine part of her life now.

However, we soon had a reality check when her back pain got worse and radiated to her opposite flank. She wondered whether she had sprained her back in the garden, and at her next chemo session she planned to discuss it with her doctors but did not get an opportunity. I was annoyed about this, but Kathleen did not want to cause a fuss and so we returned home, both in bad form. She was unable to sleep and increased her pain medication. She was sure it was a musculoskeletal problem and I reluctantly went along with her diagnosis, as I did not want to scare or upset her any more. It went from bad to worse over the following few days, and when another tooth fell out, she had had enough. After an emergency visit to her dentist, she had an MRI scan of her back that revealed a fracture of the twelfth thoracic vertebra. After much discussion among the radiologists, it was confirmed to be a benign osteoporotic fracture, the kind often related to chemotherapy treatment, rather than the feared pathological fracture from a secondary bone cancer. She was reviewed by a palliative care specialist and more pain medication was prescribed.

The garden was where Kathleen fought her pain and self-doubt. If she was able to perform in the garden, she could survive 'on the stage', in the outside world. In the first year of her illness, the pain masked the breathing problem, whereas in the second year it was the reverse. Early on she had been prescribed oral opioid analgesics for pain relief but decided not to take them. She opted to suffer rather than submit.

'If I start taking painkillers, I won't be able to continue working or to drive, or even to drink,' she complained to me one day, as we sat on the bench to admire our day's work.

I knew it was a plea for acknowledgement and support.

'Well, Mum, you are not supposed to drive and drink. I will do that and you can concentrate on working!' My double entendre often had the desired effect and she could focus again on her flowers, which were sprouting and splitting the ground ivy.

'Let's dig another hole for this plant, Dad, before it rains.'

But at a certain point, even the garden's beauty and tranquil grandeur did not ease the pain and we had to tackle the issue again. The dosage of Targin, the opiate painkiller that had been prescribed, was small and unlikely to interfere with her routine.

'I have read the leaflet, Mum, and it is a low dose and is also good for your restless leg syndrome which affects you at night.'

I knew she had also read the leaflet and was less convinced, and she only agreed to take it sporadically at first. It was a start but quickly became a footnote, as each evening she filled her stomach with a pharmacy of tablets fit for an addict. She was, however, even more reluctant to sample the transdermal patch, a slow-release similar analgesic which the palliative care physician had prescribed towards the end of the first year.

'He must think I am on the way out, and he must know more about my disease than I do,' she remarked, as she searched my eyes for any response.

'I think his idea is that with the chemo and all the tablets you are taking the oral analgesics are getting lost in your system.'

She was not buying this surgical nonsense. 'That's a stupid comment, even from you!' I did not want to remind her of all the extra, undocumented self-prescribed medicines in her bedside locker that she consumed each night.

She used her continuing garden work to prop up her case to carry on as normal. But even there, the reality of disease was inescapable and evident all year round. The weeds ensnared and clung to the healthy stems and foliage, in the manner of cancer cells, despite the best efforts of the diligent and impatient gardener.

'Mum, should I cut these heavy sagging branches with the large lumpy growths along their boughs?'

'No,' she said. 'They are apple trees and are still alive. Leave them alone.'

'It would let more light in,' I replied but there was no further discussion forthcoming on that topic, and so I left it be. Wild growth contained within boundaries and borders buys some time. And for a while, there is more order than disorder.

❖

'Who is he talking to, I wonder?' one of Leo Varadkar's entourage might have asked as he entered the Ardboyne Hotel in Navan on 31 May 2017 – just before he was elected leader of his party, and subsequently Taoiseach. Kathleen had buttonholed him on the day and they had a brief, friendly chat. She was happy to say hello and wish him well. He had once been a junior hospital doctor in Navan and he knew her. All she was doing that day was reminding him she was still around.

Kathleen knew most of the local politicians and got on well with them. They were all aware of her strong, almost territorial, commitment to the hospital, and they all sought and valued her advice and counsel. She gave these freely and was happy when they listened. While there have been gains over her working lifetime, the hospital's future is still uncertain. The new generation of consultants are not as territorial or as tolerant as she was. Their commitment to their professional vocation is their principal focus, and they don't have time for tea and buns. There is now a much greater distance between them and lay hospital management, which has created a healthier hospital working environment.

Around this time, we realised that too many things were happening and too many specialists were involved in her treatment. We both decided Kathleen needed a family doctor to coordinate her care and her medications. She also needed a colleague nearer to home she could call on at short notice and who had more time to talk and to listen to her. She was taken on by a practice run by two of her former trainees. After this had been sorted, we decided to cancel a planned holiday and take stock.

We agreed the best therapy was working in the garden together, and the unusually warm spring and summer weather in 2017 was a godsend. We also decided that, for now, she should continue with her work in the IHF, the College and with her reduced private practice. I signed up to provide her with more logistic support. Meanwhile, her newly appointed family doctor arranged for a local palliative care team to visit her at home. She had a Zometa infusion to increase her bone calcium and prepare her for three sessions of root canal treatment. However, during the course of this dental work, she developed more abdominal and flank pain, which greatly upset her. I wondered about a recurrence of diverticulitis because her abdomen was tender to palpation. After another CT scan, that particular diagnosis was confirmed (along with much else which was not reported on this occasion). This was such a relief to her, as she had already commenced her preparations for Peter and Nerea's wedding in September, and just a week earlier we had made a weekend trip to visit Nerea's family in Spain, where she bought her mother-of-the groom dress with fanfare and delight.

Our second grandchild was born two weeks later, in mid-July. We met Harry the morning after he was born in Holles Street, and later that day we returned to Connemara for our annual holiday. We spent two happy days alone in glorious sunshine, walking, swimming and picnicking on Lettergesh beach, before Ruth, Paddy and Finn arrived to share the happiness. Finn got to know Tullymore Danny and Oisín, when I pushed the buggy up close to the gap in the hedge. Unlike cows that come close to greet and can therefore be somewhat disconcerting for children, ponies stand still and stare, and so Finn could take his time to stare in turn and weigh them up at his own pace.

Kathleen and I went back to Collon for a few days for a visit to the dentist, followed by another chemo session, and then we returned to Connemara to join the annual gathering of friends there. It was during that bank holiday week she decided to write this book, after we attended the interment of the ashes of a dear friend in a cemetery overlooking the ocean. As I walked among the old headstones, I read an inscription that seemed to catch the mood of our fading life together: 'The cart is shaken all to pieces and the rugged road is at its end.'

❖

Living with cancer, for many, is a full-time occupation with no room for any other kind of work or play. In Kathleen's case, it was a disguised burden she carried along with her. But that only works if people don't know you have cancer or, if they do, are at least unaware of its nature or extent. Otherwise, the ID card, the badge that comes with it, puts more than a name to your face. The morning greeting is no longer a glance and a wave. There is more eye contact, a slightly exaggerated smile, imperceptible at first, but a week or month later, you become aware of the fleeting, furtive stare, the kind of look of recognition given to a 'lame-duck' politician. That feeling is familiar to many public servants in Ireland the day after retirement, when the employer and colleagues wish you well and then take your name off their mailing lists.

It had not come to that yet because very few knew enough about her and, like all cancer patients, her life was full of events, most of which were unpleasant but which she had managed to conceal. The busy narrative becomes the main storyline and all the turmoil has to be recorded. It is not an easy read and in truth it is likely to be glossed over by the reader. The headlines are enough. It is the commentary and review that holds the interest and attention, rather than the stark, unrelenting recitation of the unpalatable detail.

The Connemara days that year were, as usual, packed with routine and intrigue. For those few weeks in the year we had new neighbours – the settled community and the 'blow-ins'. Most of the blow-ins were from 'the East' and were well-to-do and commanding in all respects. We were from the East too, but we were from outside the Pale and thus less notable and more suited to the local quiet country lanes than the closely observed and travelled highways. Kathleen could mix and match, but I preferred to maintain my normal persona of being odd, boring and socially unpredictable, much to her annoyance!

Whether to be seen or remain unseen was the constant question. Nothing usually happens in the place until nine or ten in the morning. And you don't always have to go out to enjoy the happenings in the locality. Each large overlooking window in the house can be a sentry post that provides sample material for conversation for the day.

'Michael was up early this morning. I saw him drive up for the paper and some jam rolls – and there's Aiden and his guests going past the pier on the loop walk,' I reported to Mum.

'You don't need your shirt and vest anymore, Dad. It's time to put on your casual tops and short trousers, or else you will stand out as a nerd,' she said by way of reply.

The morning newspaper and the old-school transistor radio were the favoured sources of news in Connemara. Mobile phones and laptops had access and coverage problems, as information technology was not yet embedded in the region. Conversing with real people in the flesh using nouns, verbs and adjectives was part of the novelty of the place. The summertime regulars embraced its pace and space and customs, while retaining and exploiting their networking skills. The weather determined the day's activities. Each sunny morning Kathleen prepared the picnic lunch, which was consumed on Lettergesh beach or occasionally, as a treat for Mum, in Glassilaun, which driving-wise was a more demanding venue for Dad to navigate in his later years. On the wet days, when the rain never stopped, the day was passed in the car viewing landmarks of note and praying for a break in the clouds or, alternatively, in the front room with a large jigsaw puzzle and a pack of cards. The few accessible TV channels in our house were Irish, showing 'home fare' entertainment, decent old movies and Gaelic football and hurling matches. The local pub filled up from 6 p.m. and was where the news of every family's day was disclosed.

Attending Mass on Sundays was an important communal occasion that was good for the soul but served other purposes also. It was where you went along to see the latest arrivals to the village and, after the service, to find out what parties were being planned for the week ahead. In between, all listened earnestly to the priest as he told stories about God and Mammon. The tall tales recounted at the dinner parties were delivered with fervour and bravado. They were most often old stories embellished for effect and always greeted with approval and applause. The jokes, too, were the same as last year, and the laughter invariably broke out long before the punchline was reached. It did not matter, as the red and white had already turned the guests into a jolly and most receptive audience.

20

LOOSE ENDS

My children and I were keen to explore any new chemo or immunotherapy. My oncologist had already told me that, as my histology markers had revealed I had 'wild type' disease with few mutations, I was therefore not suitable for immunotherapy. But I wanted more tests done after reading an article in a magazine, even though I was not very hopeful. Over the last year Finbar and I had been reading a lot about immunotherapy. We had come across an article published in the journal Science *about a new drug which had dramatic beneficial effects in 86 patients with various forms of previously untreatable cancer. This involved a new approach which was based on the treatment of genetic abnormalities, rather than the primary location of the disease. This seemed to fit my diagnosis of CUP.*

Last summer after completing my first course of chemotherapy – which had not worked – I discussed possible treatment options in the US with my physician/oncologist.

He gently advised me to use my time to enjoy my new and first grandchild, born last autumn, and my two sons' upcoming weddings. This was good advice which I valued, and fortunately I remained well enough to enjoy my first grandchild's arrival and my eldest son's wedding, followed shortly afterwards by the arrival of my second grandchild, in July just past. These were wonderful events and I now look forward to my second son's wedding in Spain next month. If I get through that without any more scares, I will discuss further treatment options with Finbar but I am very grateful the Lord has spared me so far.

By the end of a happy and fulfilling summer, it was time to take stock.

'Is it time, Mum, to write to the Heart Foundation and the College and tell them you are ill and need to stop?' She had already decided not to put her name forward again for election to the council of the College.

'Let's wait until next week. They know I am having chemo.'

'Yes, Mum, but they don't know it is not working.' At this, she just waved me away, which was her usual tactic when she did not like what she was hearing or did not agree with me.

I spoke to her again about a month later, after she showed me a list she had just compiled of her jewellery and who she wanted to leave it to, with the name placed opposite each listed piece.

'They will be annoyed if they find out how bad things

are. Maybe we can send an email, alerting them that you are winding down and that they need to be making contingency plans.'

There was no dismissive wave on this occasion. 'Dad, will you draft the emails and show them to me?'

She did not want to give up, and the College and Heart Foundation were both gracious in facilitating her wishes to stay involved – but at least now they knew the score. She was delighted sometime later to see her joint letter with Tim Collins on the Public Health (Alcohol) Bill published in the *Irish Times* on 9 November.

❖

I was not sure about immunotherapy and not convinced there was enough sand left in the hourglass to consider another form of treatment. Kathleen was keener, however, and wanted to try anything new that might work. The thing about filling up the days with constant work and activity – including long-forsaken family life, which provides quality distraction – is that it comes with a downside. You lose sight of the sentence that was handed down and there is less time to plan for more time. When secondary disease is the first cancer calling card, the shock is greater, and even more so when, as with Kathleen, you have been feeling perfectly well, only to be told out of the blue you have a terminal disease. Whenever such a type of secondary cancer takes hold, it is not a gradual decline that occurs. The 'well' time is priceless and every day is counted and valued, and though often laden with suffering, it is still possible to withstand all the effects of disease and the side-effects of treatment and bounce back, which she did again and again. However, when the tipping point arrives, you fall over a cliff.

When Kathleen's GP referred her to the local palliative care team, there was a silent recognition on both our parts that the timing of this initiative was right. The palliative care team is a multidisciplinary specialty team of doctors, nurses, physiotherapists and social workers. The difference is they are not involved in finding out what's wrong with the patient: they already know what's wrong and that it cannot be fixed. There is often a transition period when both the 'curative' and palliative teams, led by the doctors, provide combined care. There is a temptation to say the patient is getting the best of both worlds at this point: in a perverse way, this period of overlap between the two teams can sometimes be a source of comfort, as in theory it allows the patient time to come to terms with his or her terminal state. In a broader sense, however, the sooner total care responsibility is transferred, the better, as the great value of the palliative team is in their expertise in preparing, assisting and supporting the patient to die with dignity.

21

TWO MORE 'WEDDINGS AT CANA', AN ANNIVERSARY AND A FINAL FLING FOR THE HEART FOUNDATION

Everything was happening in a rush now, and I knew I was running out of time. My second grandson, Harry, had been born in mid-July and I was thrilled to see him within a few hours of his birth. It was another milestone reached which meant so much to me. My second son, Peter, and his long-term girlfriend, Nerea from Logroño in Spain, got married there in September and I made it. I bought a beautiful Spanish dress and had a formal role in the marriage ceremony, which was a great boost for me and I was so grateful to be there.

A few weeks later Finbar and I returned to Spain for what we knew would be our last holiday. The trip happened by chance because we had been invited to the wedding of the son of Colm O'Morain, the doctor who diagnosed my cancer and who was one of our classmates and a long-time friend. I did not think I would be able for it but Finbar made all the arrangements just in case, and we went for it! The wedding took place in an idyllic coastal resort in Begur and we stayed on in a fancy hotel, and I had two swims in the sea and managed to finish a short mountain trek. It was a memorable happy few days and coincided with our 40th wedding anniversary, which we celebrated at dinner the evening before we returned home. We reminisced about our own wedding in University Church in St Stephen's Green in 1977, and our wedding breakfast in the famous Hibernian Hotel.

Kathleen was able to let go of the cancer and park it in another place for the few days we spent in Logroño at our second son's wedding. She managed to keep some joy and fun in reserve for the wedding celebrations, which went on for three days. She had now reached all her family milestones and ticked all her professional boxes and was ready to take her leave of the Heart Foundation and the College, knowing that her work was done.

She used to remind me that I had never written a poem about her. One of our exercises at the creative writing course I signed up to after Kathleen died was to write a short commentary about a photograph that had some special meaning and my emotional response to it. For the exercise I decided to write that poem and found by chance the one photo among hundreds that includes the two of us, as she watched me deliver my speech at Peter and Nerea's wedding.

It's all about the smile.
A snapshot suspended in time.
Happy, relaxed and active
As opposed to happy, relaxed and passive,
Which looks the same.
But not with such a pose.
The head tilt, the eyes and forearms
All responsive and engaged.
He must have just said something.
It might have been funny
But her son is not sharing the joke
So a joke was not the prompt.
Was it a 'sweet nothing' somehow shared without eye contact?
Or has his delivery to the Spanish guests
Produced a frisson of delight?
The faint ripple of his smile and his gaze
Suggest a pause in his speech.
An easy performance,
Though not quite spontaneous.
He cannot see her smile
But it has been captured
For posterity,

And more importantly, for him.
The reality is she is already dying,
And has at that very moment
Reached the final milestone
She set herself a year ago.
Only she and he know about
The fading time, and how quick
The passage of that day.
The gay and joyous abandon
Though rare and fleeting
Is very precious now.
The image, a memory etched
To ensure he soldiers on.

Begur was her last post and adieu. She had finally signalled and acknowledged her growing infirmity to me the day before we flew to Barcelona. We were heading up to the Mater for her review CT scan.

'I have got more short of breath, Dad – do you think I am fit to travel?' she said out of the blue.

'Well, you are planning to do your clinic in Navan this afternoon!' I replied.

'You know I cannot cancel the clinic at this short notice.'

'Well, I cannot cancel the trip to Begur at this stage either and I know you want to go.' I squeezed her hand and that was the end of the conversation. It was her last opportunity to live on her own terms and to lay the heavy burden down for a few precious days and dream of all the good times together. She wanted some safe, protected space to forget her troubles and after that dismissed any mention by me of her illness. She did this at some later cost, but it was worth it. I made only one, futile, intervention but was glad I did not spoil the spontaneous moments of happiness. One of these was the sea filling the private cove below our hotel room and its invitation to swim one last time, accepted by Kathleen with gratitude and pleasure; another was the expression of wonder and delight on her face as she reached a 'mountain' summit, after which we made the short descent to the nearby beach for lunch and took a taxi back to lie in the sun at the poolside. This was her earthly paradise.

On our way back home, Kathleen lost her mobile phone in Barcelona airport and was very upset. After our anniversary celebrations in Begur, it was a real let-down that she now was without her main source of communication. We bought a new phone some days later but a lot of her personal data could not be retrieved from the cloud. When David arrived home with his wedding photographs, this gave Mum a welcome lift in mood. He helped her figure out how to get some of the lost messages back from the cloud and into her new phone and was able to reconnect her to all her friends. For some reason, her texting ability improved with the new screen and emojis, but her messages were subdued and gloomy, particularly after the latest scan confirmed significant progression of the disease.

Kathleen was now more aware of her shortness of breath and her long-standing cough was becoming troublesome again. She had been on steroids intermittently for three months and was becoming dependent on them. At this point she was in a phase of denial and believed from her study of the literature that her respiratory symptoms might be due to the chemotherapy drug Gemzar. Her oncologist, Professor Des Carney, told her this was very unlikely and from that moment it seemed certain the cancer had spread to her lungs. As always, she took the mortal blow with great calmness and fortitude, but did not want to give up yet. At a subsequent meeting, Des confirmed the bad news but did not labour the message and gave us time and space to talk it through with him. In so far as is possible in this situation, it was a good interactive consultation and Kathleen was grateful to him.

As we walked out, she turned to me and, without referring to the news we had received, said, 'Let's go and get my red dress out of the car, and I will change in your office and you can drive me down to the lunch.'

There was a Heart Foundation charity lunch in town that day and she had decided to bring the dress in case she might go. Her sister Joan met her there and Kathleen remarked to her, 'I've not put a brush through my hair, no time'. When asked by her sister how she was, she simply said, 'Not good news – no more to be done!' Joan expressed surprise that she had decided to come and Kathleen responded, 'I might as well while I can.'

It summed up her resolve and her determination to fight the cancer to the bitter end.

On the drive home that evening she was in philosophical mood, wondering what the future had in store. Moving on quickly was always her way – there was no point on dwelling on the bad stuff.

'What else do I need to do, Dad?'

'Well,' I said, 'we have our anniversary celebration again on Sunday with all the family.'

'You know that will be my last one, Dad.'

'One step at a time, Mum – you still have to finish your work in the IHF and buy the new HQ and complete your hospital site reports for the College. And you have not told them much about your recent illness updates.'

'Well, maybe I should,' she replied, and then we both lapsed into silence.

Neither of us slept that night, and I repaired at 2.45 a.m. Kathleen's good friend Trish called the next morning and her mood lifted. Later that day, we spent some time together in the garden, and I attacked some of the overhanging tree branches with a ladder and a saw in order to let more sunlight in.

'Promise me you won't ever climb ladders on your own.'

It was the 'ever' in the sentence that jolted me.

'Are you worried about my osteoporosis?' I said.

'I am not joking, Dad.'

'I know,' I said. I had only recently been rescued by her

after climbing onto the high end of the inner garden wall to remove overhanging creeping ivy from the neighbour's adjoining overgrown garden. The ladder had fallen as I reached the summit and I was afraid to jump or scale down an ailing tree. I opted to sit quietly on top of some loose flat concrete blocks and wait, as darkness descended on the Collon landscape. Apart from a prowling cat who stared up at me, I was alone in my secluded garden. Eventually, after nearly two hours, she found me.

The first of October 2017 was our 40th wedding anniversary and all the children were home for it. We had a family lunch for 20 people, prepared by Sue, Kathleen's good friend from her book club. Later that afternoon Kathleen told them the latest cancer update in her own way. As she was gently breaking the news, I was aimlessly pottering about, considering how I would explain it to them. Chemotherapy works by killing cells, good ones and bad ones, but in Mum's case mainly good ones. The bad ones had been multiplying unseen and were now spreading like ivy.

Ruth, Paddy and Finn stayed on for the following week, so that we could also celebrate Finn's first birthday. Midweek, we had another early-morning drive to the Mater when Kathleen had another Zometa infusion, which was usually well tolerated. She seemed more relaxed, until unfortunately one of the junior doctors told her that her shortness of breath was due to metastatic lung disease. She was not expecting such a definitive response to a throwaway request for an opinion on respiratory symptoms. She was very upset when I collected her.

'I am finished, Dad – I may as well pack my bags.'

Open disclosure has its limitations, even when it is assumed the patient knows what is happening because she is a doctor. I was running out of non sequiturs and decided, with her agreement, to arrange an urgent consultation with a friendly respiratory physician, whom she saw next day. Reassurance always works, even in adversity. The diagnosis stays the same but the nature of the explanation and the way it is delivered can calm the frightened mind.

22

'THE CART IS SHAKEN ALL TO PIECES'

Soldiering on here with chemo – cannot find primary and no real improvement after year of Gemzar and Carboplatin. So continue same. Waiting for some magic! Shortly after I returned home from Begur I became more aware of breathlessness, wheeze and an increased heart rate. The cause could not be found though I thought at first it was allergic. My doctors thought it was cancer-related. If that is the case, I should have urgent chemo.

I counted my blessings.

Good things: was in Edinburgh for grandson's birth in October 2016. Was at David's wedding in March 2017. Harry's birth in Holles Street, July 2017. Peter's wedding in September 2017. Nice holiday in Begur at wedding of my consultant's son later that month. Helped plan, attended and participated in 50th anniversary celebrations of IHF in 2017.

Spent 25 great years on the council of the Royal College of Physicians in Ireland. Spent 31 happy and wonderful years in Our Lady's Hospital, Navan. Grandad's funeral in Warrenpoint.

Thursday 12 October 2017 was the beginning of the end. I was up at 7 a.m. Mum was in poor form. I brought breakfast to her and was then collected at 9 a.m. by my friend and walking partner Jeremy and we went off for a prearranged beach walk in Togher. When I returned at 11.30, I found Mum sitting at the computer in the library. She was in distress and very short of breath, and though she initially resisted my advice that she needed to go into hospital, she did not stop me contacting the hospital to make the necessary arrangements.

'It is in my lungs now, Dad, not good – what do you think?'

'Let us wait and get the tests done. I love you, Mum.'

She gently squeezed my hand but said no more.

We arrived in the Mater Private at 5.30 that afternoon and went to the admissions office. In the adjacent waiting room, two patients were ahead of us who appeared to me to be routine elective cases. We sat down but I was agitated – I could see that there was no one in the office and got up to go and find somebody. Kathleen told me to sit down and wait. When the admissions officer returned, I went in to see him to explain the urgency of the situation, but he did not respond with the alacrity I expected. As I returned to my seat, I could see Kathleen was upset.

'Stop that nonsense, Finbar, you are being very rude. They are busy.'

'I am sorry, Mum. I just wanted to tell him you are an urgent case.'

Within about five minutes a nurse arrived, accompanied by a porter with a wheelchair, and Kathleen was admitted to the High Dependency Unit. A CT scan confirmed a very significant pulmonary embolus. We were both surprised at the diagnosis, expecting instead that it was likely to reveal an extension of the cancer to her lungs. Ultimately, it did show that also, but the acute event was the pulmonary embolus.

It was a barn-door case, and we should have known it. When we were in Begur in Spain three weeks earlier, I had noticed a swelling in one of her legs. When I brought it to her attention, she dismissed my concern that it signalled a DVT, telling me it was a common occurrence with her after a long day on her feet and it would resolve after she rested and elevated her legs. I did not argue with her at the time and accepted her explanation, but in retrospect it was a harbinger of impending trouble. By this time, we had both had our fill of medical interventions, and each chose to stay a little longer in denial mode. Unfortunately, now the clot had had its devastating say when it travelled to her right main pulmonary artery (MPA).

More disaster – pulmonary embolus, Right MPA – dyspnoea [laboured breathing] occurring on therapeutic Innohep. I have a thrombophilia, and of course a cancer patient has increased risk of clot in any case, also in last three weeks my mobility has reduced – another risk factor. In my case, the 'full Monty' applied!

We came to MPH [Mater Private Hospital] at around 5 p.m. CT PA – pulmonary embolus – admitted to ICU under the care of expert and kind respiratory physician. Decision to change to BD Clexane [another anticoagulant drug]. Hope it works. I have major problems: three months' history of cough, stridor [loud, laboured breathing] and bronchospasm. I had thought this was asthma, an allergy, but my oncologist thinks it is cancer related, possibly lymphangitis carcinomatosis, which is a disaster. Will I have more chemo? Already two failed chemo regimes. What to do? I should put it off, as I am not fit after a massive pulmonary embolus. The 'Honour's case' was becoming more difficult to manage!

What if we had paid more attention to the swollen leg three weeks earlier? She was always careful about her prescribed medications and since commencing chemotherapy always took her daily Innohep injections. Maybe if she had reported the leg swelling to her doctor after returning from Spain, an ultrasound scan would have confirmed the presence of a clot in her leg, and the anticoagulant could have been changed or the dose of Innohep increased. But we did not further engage in this 'what if' conversation, as it served no useful purpose. I arrived home tired that evening at about 10 p.m., swallowed my warfarin tablets and went to bed.

22:23
F: *Home Mum. Miss you. Love Dad.*

22:56
F: *Mum, are you OK? Did not hear back from last text. Love Dad.*

23:02
K: *In stepdown 2nd floor, stable. No one in bed with me! xx*

23:03
K: *Vitals stable! xx*

23:04
F: *Am home in your bed with myself! xxx*

23:05
K: *Xxx*

23:07
F: *You must be in bed on your own if your vitals are stable!*

Around this time we were both beginning to understand our lonely plight, as a couple, but also now as two loving companions inevitably moving apart and heading in different directions. I spent more time walking about on my own in Dublin, trying to make sense of what was happening to us. One frequent port of call was Trinity College, where I was able to pace about with a sure, confident step. My nondescript appearance in a long tweed overcoat and woolly hat attracted no attention from the tutors and professors wandering by, scarcely distinguishable themselves among the constant stream of students. Trinity is a meeting place, a thoroughfare, a short cut to Pearse Street and Nassau Street. Its buildings' façades observe the moving maze of people without acknowledgement or interest. My visits were mostly silent trips, with facial expressions and hand movements my only interactions with the passing crowd before I slipped away. The beggar, busker and down-and-out were going about a similar journey in their own sphere of influence somewhere nearby. So too were the banker, civil servant and shopper. I stopped at times to reflect on where I fitted in this urban landscape. Was I an isolated figure or part of some set piece, moving on and off a stage? The backdrop of an old historic city, a famous university and a diverse sample of 21st-century society raises many questions but the only one that mattered to me at that time was how long she would last. Is there some order in this chaos? Are we all interdependent? Do we have a part to play, a story to tell

THE HEAVENS ARE ALL BLUE

and are we all on the same stage? Is there really somebody up there looking after us? Suddenly, I recalled the inscription on the headstone in Connemara. It was like a familiar tune in my head — 'this cart is shaken all to pieces and the rugged road is at an end'.

After the daydream, it was back to the real world. During the month Kathleen was an inpatient in the Mater, I often paused to browse the newspapers on my walk back up O'Connell Street to the hospital. The front page of the *Herald* frequently had some tale of woe in bold headlines about an incident that had occurred in the city centre. The characters involved had probably passed by me the day before.

The incidence of pulmonary embolism in the US is estimated at 1 per 1000. It is a common cause of death in hospitalised patients. The diagnosis is often missed. Now, with the use of routine thrombo-prophylaxis [preventive action against abnormal clotting] with low molecular weight Heparin, the death rate has reduced. In my case because of my risk factors, I was already on full dose, therapeutic low molecular weight Heparin, and therefore presented a difficult management challenge to the medical staff. About 10 per cent of patients who develop a pulmonary embolus die t in the first hour, though anticoagulation therapy has reduced this to 5 per cent.

It was the night before Storm Ophelia, and I was fortunately promptly diagnosed with a pulmonary embolus following a CT angiogram. My clever doctors decided to change and increase the dose of my anticoagulation medicine to ensure the clot did not extend further, as it had already reached the right main pulmonary artery and had created a life-threatening condition. This was a very worrying development for me and my doctors/all of us. To help relieve my anxiety, my son Peter rigged up an iPad in the ICU with earphones and I watched a movie – The Notebook – *surrounded by medical machines and monitors. The other very sick patients in the unit were not sure what to make of it all!*

I wondered at the time if I should elect not to be resuscitated in the event that I had a cardiac arrest. The combination of this very serious complication and my advanced underlying cancer meant my prognosis was grim. I had often jokingly said in recent times that a quick, painless pulmonary embolus might be a great exit strategy, given my cancer diagnosis! However now that it appeared a distinct possibility, I decided not to mention it [the question of resuscitation] just yet; to take my chances and see what my doctors came up with to manage an 'Honour's case' like mine. At any rate I survived the first week, with the prospect of indefinite twice daily anticoagulant injections ahead of me. My computer-literate family arranged more movie iPad distraction and mentally I stayed on track.

Gemzar, Herceptin, FOLFOX, Pembro; oncology wards; low white cell and platelet counts; nausea, vomiting and diarrhoea – this is the familiar language of the cancer patient. Such language features in everyday conversations at home in the towns and villages of Ireland. It spells trouble wherever it is spoken, and the resultant fear and uncertainty it evokes spreads beyond the family and into the local community. But not all cancer patients are dying anymore: many are now 'well cancer patients', who are getting more targeted and refined treatment and often respond to it and get better. They share the day wards with the 'sick cancer patients' – those receiving palliative chemotherapy who do poorly and are often easy to spot among their peers because they are very much fewer in number and look unwell, even to the untutored eye. Some of them will be missing next time round, and the regulars with their newly acquired 'clinical acumen' will silently wonder about their fate. This is an unnerving experience and can shake everyone's confidence, as the demons always seem to be in the room – but this is a false perception. While cancer is increasing in incidence, it is a more benign disease today than it ever has been because it is being diagnosed early, before it becomes invasive. And so the full and overflowing cancer day wards no longer define your destiny. Instead they are becoming beacons of hope and recovery for many – and, thankfully, less fertile ground for memoirs!

Chemotherapy is a poison and is best used in 'healthy' patients with 'good' cancers who can tolerate its toxicity, in the knowledge they are likely to do well and respond. Most are treated as day cases and receive their infusions over a few hours and go home. They don't get sick in the day wards – that will happen when they get home and the side-effects of the chemo kick in. The medicine works on the wards, whereas the poison works in the home. The longer patients can be treated in the day ward, the better chance they have of a good outcome. When their scheduled treatment session is deferred because their haemoglobin, white blood cells or platelets are low, or they need to be admitted to a hospital bed, this means the poison is working at least as well as the medicine. If the advance of the disease has been halted or reversed, the medicine wins and life is prolonged, the disease stabilised, and, increasingly, remission is achieved. This will be greeted with great relief and joy, and the doctor will be praised. The losses, on the other hand, are always due to the disease, and the only comeback is to try again.

The sick cancer patients usually present with significant symptoms and often have advanced disease at diagnosis. They are clinically unwell at the outset and become sicker with chemotherapy, which rarely works for them – though, unfortunately, it takes time before that is clearly evident and acknowledged. The only object of the treatment for many of these patients is to buy some time but that comes at a cost of agony to the mind and body. Also a very small number of cases with advanced disease present with no significant symptoms; for them, chemotherapy is the only conventional form of treatment available but it rarely works. Whether it buys some time is moot. In that situation you are at the cliff edge and about to fall over. You stay reasonably well for a time and then things happen. One leg swells, then you get short of breath climbing stairs and lose your appetite and then you fall over the cliff. Kathleen was in this latter group but that only fully dawned on us a long way down the line.

The relentless and often silent suffering caused by chemotherapy is described with anguish in all the cancer memoirs. No one has a good word to say about it, but they all endure it and its side-effects and describe them in visceral, painful language; they accept the suffering in the hope of a cure. Christopher Hitchens and Donald Hall encapsulate it so well in their writing: 'Today, she looked at her bald head and at her face swollen with Prednisone'; 'Worst of all is chemo-brain. Dull and stuperous'; 'On a much too regular basis, the disease serves me up a flavour of the month. It might be random sores and ulcers, on the tongue or in the mouth …'

The perversity of the cure being worse than the disease is a feature in all such memoirs. This consistent and universal data trumps the requirement to conduct a double-blind study, and surely should spur on the search for personalised target treatment for all cancer patients. Today's last-resort treatment options such as immunotherapies should be provided in some cases as first-line treatments, with chemotherapy relegated to last-resort status. For the CUP cases like Kathleen's, the goal must be to find the primary and to continue the search throughout the course of treatment. The standard response from the doctor – that 'It does not matter where the primary is, you already have secondary disease' – should be consigned to the dustbin. While you are above ground, the clock is the calendar and the days are full of hope. One more day gone, one less to go is universal and so there is no time to lose.

16 October 2017

After two failed chemos, what to do? In today's Irish Times, *'Breaking a Taboo' – the results of a survey by the Irish Hospice Foundation – makes interesting reading for me. It highlights people's concerns around end-of-life issues. Most people surveyed want to be pain-free and to die at home. Speakers at the conference launching the survey said that up to a third of terminally ill patients receive inappropriate chemotherapy and inappropriate cardio-pulmonary resuscitation, and 42 per cent are admitted to intensive care units. Judge Catherine McGuinness, a recently retired Supreme Court Judge, urged the introduction of a 'Think Ahead' document to record patient care preferences. I now have an increased number of bulky pulmonary nodes causing respiratory symptoms but my 'performance status' is fair. How far to go with treatment? Should I discuss this with my doctors or leave it to them to decide? I am not sure of end-of-life thoughts ...*

❖

How close is death?
The train stops at every station.
Will she be OK as long as it is moving?
What happens when it reaches its destination and the engine is switched off?
Perhaps she leaves the train to start another journey.
In that case there is no need to answer the questions.

23

LAST ROLL OF THE DICE AND END OF DAYS

Bad diagnosis. Immunotherapy last roll of dice, and then? Time to think of next life. Main concerns are pain and breathing. Palliative care services assure me symptoms can be relieved. Would hospice care be better and less stressful for family? Hospice Report/Dignitas/The Right to Die – should it be legal? Dr Regina McQuillan [Chairperson of the Irish Association for Palliative Care] says she can see some people might feel pressure to go this route. I wonder should it be available as an option? Perhaps if people don't want to be a huge burden, that option should be available to them. In my case I could decline medical treatment, e.g. anticoagulants for thrombosis, antibiotics for sepsis.

So, the books say that after anger comes acceptance – I have not reached that yet. Religion would help. I am most concerned about symptom control, and how will Finbar cope.

October 2017

Texting is only way I can keep in touch with the outside world. 'Thanks A. So sorry for late response. Was hoping to make wedding but health not progressing as well as hoped!' 'M. Clot improving slightly. Reading blog of cancer sufferer Emma Hannigan – all to live for – hilarious so far!' 'Thanks M. Woe is me, hoping for miracle!' 'J. Thank you for lovely books. Fortunately my eyes still work and so I can enjoy. Back against wall now.'

When I look back on her contemporaneous records, I become upset and emotional because I thought I was protecting her from the agonies of cancer. To some extent I was, but my efforts were largely concentrated on her physical suffering. Little did I realise that she was shielding me from her mental anguish, which was a much more fearsome burden, the more so as she knew the inevitable outcome from early on. Of course, I knew too, but I tried to fend it off by not openly acknowledging or discussing it with her. My mindful approach was to deal with that distress by gentle, reassuring vocal distractions and facial emoji gestures. I believed at the time that they did help her, but now I wonder.

I feel safe in bed at night
safe from death,
as any sudden pain or ache

if it comes in darkness
is cushioned by my tired senses.
Will my half-shut eyes
see the wringer in the dew
or my only working ear
Hear the tolling bell?
Probably not, best forgotten.

The oxygen man arrived at the house early on 24 October, the day Kathleen was due to come home from the Mater. He installed a 'machine' in her bedroom and another in a downstairs room, with a long extension tube to enable her to walk about in some comfort. He began to explain to me how they worked. 'Just show me how to turn them on and off – I know how they work,' I said in a gentle and polite manner. She was discharged at lunchtime, with a portable device for use in transit.

On leaving the hospital, we passed one of the new electric cars, sitting in its dock and hitched up by a cable to what looked like a parking meter. It was being charged up at rest so it did not run out of energy while in motion.

'That's what I need now to keep me going!' Kathleen remarked with a wan smile.

On the way home we collected a nebuliser from the local health centre and all her meds in the pharmacy in Navan. She was exhausted by the time we got to the house. I turned on the bedroom oxygen tank while she applied her mask before settling down to rest for the afternoon. I did the household chores and cooked the supper. She came downstairs and we had our meal together in the kitchen. We watched TV and I went up to bed before her, put on her bedside light, lay down and waited.

I heard her slowly climbing the stairs and coming into the room. She was still able to put on her night dress slowly but unaided. I did not stir or look up but I was wide awake. When she got into bed, I hugged her and then she sat up with her Kindle and started to read. She rubbed the back of my legs with both her feet. This continued for a while in silence. It was a loving gesture, and also provided some symptomatic relief for her restless legs. I quickly became aware of the thin whistling noise in her nose. She suddenly asked me if I could hear it. I did not answer directly — what could I say? — and instead gently squeezed her tummy and made a humming sound of acknowledgement. I could also hear her rapid, laboured breathing, about which she remained silent.

After another short while she said it was time to take her tablets. She had a full stock of prescribed medications that she had placed in full view on the dressing table, and her own self-prescribed medicines that she had accumulated over the years were stored in her bedside locker. She took her night-time doses from the dressing table and the bedside locker, including her anticoagulant injection, leaving the 'Zimos', as she called her trusty Zimovane sleeping pills, for later. She asked me to find her inhaler and then took three puffs and an extra one, 'to be sure!' I suggested she should have some oxygen also, to which she agreed.

'I am bunched, Dad, it is the end. Not being able to breathe is the worst symptom to have. Woe is me.'

I held back tears, squeezed her tightly and then cried in silence. She placed her hand on my arm in sympathy. I composed myself, sat up and uttered what was now a well-worn refrain. 'We are going to hang in there together, Mum, and keep going.'

She smiled, signalling agreement, and resumed her reading, with a fierce determination that the cancer would not rob her of that only remaining pleasure. At about 2 a.m., she turned to me and said, 'It is time to repair.' I got up and went over to my own room to sleep. That first-night-home routine was repeated on many occasions during the subsequent short periods she spent in the house in Collon.

November 2017

I was about one week post last chemo (Gemzar) session, and I felt very bad and weak. Had I another clot? So I went back to Mater for repeat CT/pulmonary angiogram. The result – the clot had resolved, but the bad news was worse: further spread of metastatic lung disease with lymphangitis carcinomatosis [cancerous nodes in the lymph glands of the lungs]. To me in my previous life, this indicated 'curtains' for the patient! This finding explained the increased heart rate and difficult breathing.

So what now? We had sent the original histology slides to Oncologica, and we received a result which indicated a 10 per cent uptake. Is this score enough to make the disease susceptible to immunotherapy? Also, there is difficulty about accessing the drug. In the meantime my steroids, analgesics and diuretics increased. I cannot be on steroids as well as immunotherapy – a dilemma. Admitted to hospital again. Not able for visitors: cough worse and hoarse. So need papers, videos. Pat supervising portrait painting.

After the chemotherapy had reduced her host defences, it was the conventional medicines that finished her off. Clexane, Inderal, Zimovane, Nexium, Dexamethasone, Dioctyl, Ativan, Singulair, Relvar, Ventolin, Tramadol, Dymista, Becotide, Valoid, Zovirax, Augmentin, Mycostatin, Calcichew, OxyNorm, Targin.

Kathleen's above review in her diary was a good summary of her case at the time. It described a patient with terminal disease, staring into the abyss and still seeking answers and comfort. Unusually for a case review, it was presented by the patient herself and her level of insight was remarkable. It had been Kathleen's initiative to contact Oncologica, a UK-based laboratory and clinic, requesting that a sample of her original biopsy tissue be tested to see if there was a chance she might respond to immunotherapy. Her oncologist did not object, and so the forms were completed and the tissue sent.

Her clinical summary of her case was to put it up to her oncology team to assess her sympathetically for further treatment. Meanwhile she valiantly attempted to resume whatever productive life she had left and the gainful pursuits that had sustained her. She started painting at home late on in her illness and was self-taught, but she acknowledged the guidance and direction received from her sister Pat. She seemed able to enter a peaceful zone with her brush or pencil, where she was oblivious to the surrounding noise. Occasionally she would spend hours completing a picture, while engaging in a mechanical conversation with Pat.

'Now, Pattie, should we start with the background or the figures?'

Pat would take her cue: 'What about a bit of shading on the waistcoat?'

'A bit of shading on the waistcoat,' Kathleen would murmur, and then proceed to do her own thing!

As her illness progressed on its downward course, that steely application during the painting hours seemed to silence her coughing and shortness of breath and dispel their suffocating presence for a time. She also began sorting out the multiple clothes collections she had assembled over 30 years. Many outfits had their labels and price tags in place and had never been worn. She put some aside for later distribution to Ruth and her two sisters. With my assistance, she kept in email contact with the College and the IHF. She hung on to her mind and wits long after her body had failed her and so was able to continue to give advice and direction to colleagues who were unaware how frail she was.

I know this is probably the 'last roll of the dice'. I remember giving this diagnosis to patients in the past – lymphangitis carcinomatosis – and knowing how serious it was (end-stage disease). Still some little hope for immunotherapy. My oncologist at the Mater, Des Carney, trying to access drug – expensive and my diagnosis not currently part of drug trials. I am sure Des and David Fennelly [the cancer specialist at St Vincent's to whom Kathleen was referred for the immunotherapy] will be doing their best for me and I also realise my case is quite a stressor for both of them. Des has been wonderful, with great common sense; always focused on me getting the best out of the time I have left and trying not to make me too sick.

So I am waiting to hear plan. Waiting is a major part of cancer treatment – waiting for results, waiting for beds, waiting for drugs, always waiting. Hopefully news about immunotherapy in the morning. The children have read about 'Pembro' [Pembrolizumab, a drug used in immunotherapy], and probably have unrealistically high hopes.

The doctor–patient relationship requires a delicate balance between the sciences and the humanities, which challenges the art of interactive engagement and dialogue with patients to its limits. Shared decision-making between doctor and patient is the objective of medical care management. It was always so, but rarely acknowledged or practised. Over the years not much has changed in the doctor–patient power balance and the fault, if any, rests with both parties to the contract. In recent decades there has been a momentum shift to empower the patient, and all the established stakeholders have come out in support of this 'novel' approach. Whether it is correct and effective is debatable, in my view.

There is a particular dilemma in cancer care if the doctor's values and directive clinical advice are imposed, albeit unwittingly, on the patient. This is relevant when the effectiveness of treatments is often overstated, the benefits modest and the side-effects severe. The risk to the power balance is much greater, as the loss of autonomy by the patient has to be carefully factored into the doctor's management plan. Part of the default care plan is sometimes to lie and languish in bed until somebody decides what to do next. The patient has a greater chance of exerting influence when sitting or standing beside or opposite the doctor, which allows easy eye contact and thus is more conducive to a conversation between equals. Getting out of bed before the doctor comes on his or her rounds sends an important signal that reduces the gulf separating physician and patient. Fortunately, Kathleen was able to stay in conversation with her doctors until the end, and this brought out the best in them.

The PD-L1 tumour proportion score measures the likely effectiveness of the immunotherapy drug on the tumour tissue. The higher the score, the more likely it will work and induce a positive response. The score in Kathleen's case indicated a small positive response. It was sufficient to meet the criteria in the trials. However, the cut-off for a positive response varies in different trials and is very wide, and while a case could be made for Pembro, one of the checkpoint inhibitor immunotherapy drugs, it was a long shot at best. When Kathleen received the report, she phoned the clinical director of the laboratory and both of us spoke to him. His opinion was communicated to us with an air of confidence. He said that she might benefit from Pembro. It was not surprising that his encouraging tone of voice was sufficient to sway her, though the objective evidence for its efficacy with her particular diagnosis was fairly flimsy. The problem with anti-cancer medications is that even a small benefit is sufficient to promote its value. In any case, we both decided to embrace this last chance and set about trying to negotiate the remaining obstacles.

While she had known in advance that chemotherapy was going to be difficult to tolerate, looking back over her journal entries later, I was shocked at her level of insight that the toxic treatment she was enduring was futile. There was always a flicker of hope in her reflections for some 'miracle response', but after two courses of chemotherapy extending over a year she believed this would not be forthcoming, signalling an acknowledgement that medicine had run its course. While deep-down she realised that she had reached the end of the road when it came to conventional medicine, some part of her needed to at least give the immunotherapy a chance anyway. Paradoxically, she wanted to try every possible 'cure' before accepting that the medical route had nothing more to offer her in terms of time or benefit. She was more hopeful that symptomatic treatment and palliative medicine would provide at least some relief from her respiratory symptoms. On that score, sadly, she was also to be disappointed. At the end, she placed her trust in her faith to provide some light and succour to prepare her to 'cross the river'.

When I reflect now on my own daily diary entries from 2017, it is clear that each day was a trial for her. She knew she had somehow to endure her symptoms. They were not going away and she was not going to get better. I search for the good days. They occurred when she was busy with meetings and professional work or when there was a pleasant distraction. I was living each day with her and I managed well in real time, but there was a lot of doom and gloom about. I find myself still searching the diary over and over for the elusive silver linings she set so much store by, in the hope that more good days will turn up the next time I look.

Christmas Eve, 2017

I am an inpatient in SVPH [St Vincent's Private Hospital] with lymphangitis carcinomatosis and am due treatment with Nivo [Nivolumab, an immunotherapy drug]. DC and DF have gone to great lengths to try this last-chance treatment for me. They have been wonderful. It brings it back to me the great potential doctors have to do good. A letter from Ultan Daly, one of my own patients, also reminded me of this today. Doctors should be resourced and encouraged at every turn when they seek to do good. Some clinical heads with common sense should provide advice and oversight. I admire Professor Michael Barry, who goes on TV to defend the HSE policy on introducing and funding new drugs. Drug companies must be asked to produce drugs at less cost.

The early evenings in the hospital were the most difficult times to manage. Everything slowed down, even time. Her appetite was gone but she insisted on going through the motions over the supper tray. The three-course meal often stretched to over 30 minutes. Five minutes was needed to help her out of bed and seat her beside the trolley table and then adjust the oxygen line. Her routine was to pick at the fish or the chicken and then at the wobbly jelly and ice cream, which were constant dishes at both lunch and supper. She always made an effort to swallow a morsel and then pushed the plate aside. The tray was always packed on arrival and the main course would be spread over and fill the plate. Even when she managed to eat something, there was no way of knowing she was making inroads because of the size of the portion. Gentle urgings to try and eat more would fail because of her agitation and discomfort. Sipping some milk or orange juice through a straw sometimes worked. After helping her back into bed, a further attempt to encourage her to eat was made. When the tray was removed from the room, I would often fetch a new tub of ice cream, which she sometimes ate. The third course was the tea and biscuits. It was no surprise that after one or two sips the remainder in the cup was left untouched, because even in healthy times that had always been one of her calling cards!

Even as she was fading away in front of me, she didn't get old. In many respects, she carried on as normal. When she was unable to lie down anymore in her nightly bath in Collon to relax and signal the end of another busy day, she forced herself to sit on a hospital shower seat to complete her routine ablutions after a day of pain and anguish. Ruth, Joan or Pat would help her change and dress, while I kept watch on the slightly open bathroom door and the snaking oxygen line that followed her in to keep her alive. All I could do was say a silent prayer.

24

'IT IS STRANGE ...'

In spite of my doctors' trojan work, I don't feel it is going to work for me. I have had two 'goes' of Nivo, but am clinically deteriorating. So I am now thinking of the positive things in my life that I will miss.

My wonderful husband, Finbar, has been such a friend and partner over 40 years. He has been such a good husband and father to our four wonderful children, and so strong since I received this dreadful diagnosis. He could not have been more supportive and daily I thank God for the love and devotion he has given me. Our Ruth is such a wonderful girl and I am so blessed to have her as a daughter, and she is so helpful to me now. Our three boys have also been brilliant and we are so proud of them. I know they will all support their dad when I am gone. We have been blessed with two fantastically gorgeous grandsons. I have also been blessed to have been able to attend Peter's wedding to our darling Nerea, and also to have met kind and beautiful Karina,

Stephen's girlfriend from Brazil. My own family have been a tower of strength, and particularly Pat by introducing me to art, as this has provided great distraction and therapy for me in recent weeks.

This reflection does not mean that I don't terribly regret and rage that this has happened to me, and I am still wrestling with it. I am scared and worried about how the respiratory symptoms will be dealt with. I hope the Lord awaits me, along with my parents, Dr Sothy and Eilish O'Brien.

'Dad, I don't want to be buried beside people I don't know,' she said to me out of the blue.

'Well, you will be buried beside me,' I replied.

'You know what I mean,' was her anxious response.

'Yes, I do, Mum.' She was visibly relieved.

That was as much as we openly said about the existential matter. Any further verbal communications in this regard were exchanged in code. It was a few days after Christmas, and I stayed overnight on a bunk bed in her hospital room. She did not sleep because she could hardly breathe and was constantly agitated and unable to get into a comfortable position. I did not sleep because I was trying to help her to breathe and to comfort her. I also knew that night that she was crying out to tell me she was still alive.

Dying in this way is lonely and slow. The routine of Kathleen's life was gone, though she fought constantly to retain some elements of it, including, as I have said, having her nightly wash. She did not want the nurse to help her because she wanted to keep some autonomy. Earlier that evening, I had assisted her out of bed and onto the shower seat in the en suite bathroom. I turned up the oxygen flow concentration for the few minutes she was under the stream of water of the shower, and when she called, I helped her put on her nightdress. I moved the seat to the washbasin and she brushed her teeth and combed her hair. She was pleased that evening that she was able to complete her nightly routine again.

After getting back into bed she said, 'You better turn the oxygen back down, Dad. I read somewhere that too much oxygen is bad for you.'

I held back from a smart retort. 'Well, what about a cup of tea, Mum?'

I tried to be there most of the winter evenings from mid-December onwards. Usually it was Ruth who helped her through this routine and I could see that made her happy, but I knew it was a great effort for her on each occasion. Ruth was Mum's very best friend and they relied so much and for so long on each other. Now and then over the previous few weeks, Kathleen had asked me how her hellebores were faring – but I knew it was her way of reminding me of our joint commitment to the maintenance of the garden. It had lost its minders, and many of its winter flowers were also clinging to life.

With each passing day, our precious moments alone grew shorter as she needed more medical and nursing assistance. The brief interludes were filled with holding hands and physical gestures of intimacy, part of life's routine in slow motion. From her there were frowns, grimaces and gasps for breath, with occasional smiles to comfort me. They did not come easy amidst the effort to stay alive. I could not sit still and fidgeted about, trying to stay useful and engaged. I concentrated on maintaining eye contact with her so that she did not have to fend for herself or feel alone, though I knew she had already entered that latter space. Nonetheless, she was still bravely keeping a watchful eye on me and passing on subliminal messages that my job was not yet done; that when she shortly passed on the baton, she expected me to complete the race. She was still able to talk but reserved her laboured words to convey her simple needs for symptomatic relief and rest, and to tell me more than once that she loved me.

In her final few weeks, most of which were spent in hospital, Kathleen would often greet me when I entered her room with a plea: 'Talk to me; tell me what you have been doing!' Talking, particularly small talk, was never my forte, and in those months it was difficult on many occasions to know what to say. We both knew she was dying yet we clung to hope and prayer – that some change in fortune might happen or that the new treatment might work and buy us more time. It was good she had Ruth, who was a near constant presence, and so many friends who did talk endlessly to her and distract her from the burden of her illness, which could not be disguised in her interactions with me. She was still struggling to understand and rationalise why this worst-case cancer diagnosis struck without warning and at a stage beyond any prospect of conventional cure. She leaned on me to provide some semblance of an explanation, which led to a journey from medicine to metaphysics to poetry.

Confused soul is winging away
from tortured body wracked in pain.
As no breath left from long lost lungs,
it's surely time to go.

Kathleen was told she had advanced disease from the outset and that the objective of treatment was to slow its progression. She was handed a losing card on day one, and we had to make do. She was at least spared some of the related torment and mental anguish as the doctors managing her illness were able, as they cared for her, to deploy both the sciences and the 'humanities', by which I mean the art of being humane and compassionate. I have always believed that in the treatment of patients, the latter is more important and is all about individual human interaction and kind attention. It necessitates focused one-on-one time between doctor and patient, which unfortunately is in very short supply in the delivery of medical care today.

Coping with an unknown deadly illness involves managing fear, solitude and loneliness, and doctors and carers have some responsibility to be active participants in helping the patient to deal with this aspect of their suffering. Kathleen was fortunate in this regard partly because over time she came to terms with her losing battle; at the same time she never gave up the fight for some slice of luck or miracle. To get by, she combined everlasting hope with muted resignation. She was greatly assisted in her struggle to accept her fate by the local palliative care team, particularly by Dr Aisling O'Gorman and Nurse Catherine Rogers, who were able to tell her when the time came that the cancer had outpaced the medicine. They gently steered her to a place where she did not want to go. At this point, now that all her defences were down, she was able to discuss and talk it through with them until she had arrived at the station, and accepted she had to make the final preparations for her departure.

She was exercised throughout her illness by the same overarching questions: 'Why did it happen to me, and what did I do wrong?' For me, her loving partner, the answer to that question is spiritual, and finding an explanation of some kind before you die is very important; belief in God is the only fallback and relief available. Fortunately for Kathleen, that sense of consolation came early enough to allow her to die peacefully and with dignity.

Doctors are always trying to make sense of life and death. In medical practice, death is always close by and they must deal with it. While it may be relatively easy and manageable when it actually happens, many have difficulty handling it when it is near. Even doctors have a fear of death and this age-old taboo subject is often ignored despite its inevitability. There is however a reasonable expectation that the doctor is aware and understands the mindset of the dying patient, and will also help manage the denial, anger, resentment and depression that is often present.

In the ever-busier world of medicine today, it is easy to give less attention and care to the dying patient when the very opposite is required. This is never intentional and often occurs by default. Oncologists, surprisingly, are often better managing and caring for dying patients when all the chemo has been delivered and the treatment options are exhausted. Relieved of the constant burden to cure, the medicines dispensed with, their humanity can take centre stage and they can lower their professional guard to enable them to complete the contract with the patient. Because of their huge workload, their limitations come at the beginning after the diagnosis is made and during the chemo treatment, when they sometimes have insufficient time to listen and explain, and may be perceived by some patients as being too busy and rushed in their work. It is not productive to commence oncology ward rounds at 7.00 a.m., when patients are not fully alert or awake and able to engage sensibly with their doctor. Patients frequently forget most of what is said at the best of times – and nearly all that is said before breakfast!

The introduction of palliative care teams has been the biggest advance in the management algorithm of the dying patient and has enabled acceptance and a peaceful end for many.

The treating doctor is faced with many dilemmas in talking to the dying patient. How much or how little to say, and when? There is a place in the final phase of the illness for little or no conversation, when the doctor's simple supportive presence, however fleeting, at the patient's bedside is often sufficient. This serves to allay anxiety and provide reassurance and comfort, not only to the patient who may be unaware of the doctor's presence, but more significantly, to the partner and family at the bedside.

❖

On the night of New Year's Eve, Kathleen was unable to cope with her breathing difficulties and asked the nurse to phone her consultant and request that he increase her steroids. She was extremely reluctant to bother him on that particular night and was adamant with us that if it wasn't possible to reach him, she did not want anyone to make a fuss about it to the medical team. She told me the following morning that she had been embarrassed 'to interrupt his evening, as he was at a party'. This was an overreaction, but it was her nature to have such a sense of propriety and courtesy, and it was remarkable she was able to maintain such a sense of decorum in her final hours. She also expressed upset to me that she had put such pressure on both of her consultant oncologists to prescribe the Nivo, in the end to no avail. 'Don't worry about that, Mum, I wanted you to have it,' I assured her. She smiled quizzically at me and squeezed my hand.

Kathleen's voyage of discovery in her final months was portrait painting, which she took up first at home and then in hospital. It was the only 'drug' that worked, unlike the prescribed tablets she swallowed morning and evening to please her doctors. It was a means of maintaining her autonomy, of knocking medicine off its pedestal and finding another way to define her worth. With the sketchbook in front of her and a pencil in hand, she was able to focus completely. It was interesting at times to observe her in hospital as she worked on brushstrokes – how her coughing would cease and her breathing settle, and she'd appear to be at peace and away in a world of her own.

The well-worn phrase 'I love you' never lost its meaning for us, and we always signed our texts with love and kisses and smiley faces. They were part of a language of mutual reassurance and companionship that helped us to battle on. We gave up early, however, on that other well-known phrase, 'No need to worry – things will work out'. We chose to rely on, and place our faith in, love and smiley faces.

During her last week, thoughts of death were on her lips and in the air, but any words she used to express them were carefully chosen to spare any distress for me and our family. She was intent on passing on her wishes about what should happen next and used her sisters as a conduit to spread the word. She knew I would deal with everything but that I would need assistance, and it was very important to her that there was consensus about her parting requests. While I was not aware of all the manoeuvres that were afoot at the time, I can see post hoc that Kathleen had factored my 'surgical ex cathedra gene', and the fact that I was used to being in charge, into her calculations!

Her father, 'Grandad', had used the word 'protocol' when describing an agreed family plan, and now it came into use again among her sibs. About a week before she died, she told Joan, who had called to the hospital to visit, to look out the window at two jet streams in the sky in the shape of a cross. 'Look,' she said, 'it's a sign.' A few days later, she asked Joan to help me organise the funeral. She asked that the same undertakers 'who did such a good job for Granny and Grandad' be requested to make all the necessary arrangements. She wanted to be buried in Dublin and asked Joan's advice on a possible place, to which Joan replied that there was a new cemetery near her house. When Kathleen asked if it was nice, Joan said it was green and near the mountains. 'That's great, then,' was her reply. The day before she died, she asked Joan, 'Well, are we all agreed with the protocol?'

Kathleen took her last breath at 11.32 p.m. on 5 January 2018. We knew it was coming, as her long and laboured breathing had suddenly changed to quiet, gentle gasps, and within moments she was gone. It had been an exhausting day for her, and once the heavy sedation had been administered and taken hold about midday, she had crossed the road and lost earthly contact with us. All her children and siblings watched over and protected her throughout her final hours with a fierce sense of duty and gratitude. We watched her struggle to stay alive throughout the day and long into the evening. She was not going to give up without an almighty fight. Her resilience, courage and fortitude – all lifelong emblems of her character – shone through and set the bar at a higher notch for the rest of us.

I had been in early with her that morning before the nightshift ended and could see that she had had another difficult night. She started that day by thanking her night nurse for her care and attention. I could detect a change in her attitude, and it only struck me later that it was a steely determination to put some order on this day that would ensure her dignity was preserved to the last. Her consultant, David Fennelly came early, not long after I did, and spoke to her about her condition. I was sitting at the bedside as he arrived and, once again, noted his calm and reassuring manner and, in particular, the sense of duty and care he displayed in being happy to stay as long as necessary to respond to her concerns. It was a conversation between friends and peers. She was fully alert and aware that there was clinical business to discuss, but her overriding wish was to thank him and his medical and nursing colleagues for their devoted care of her. That was her signature characteristic, her gratitude for any act of kindness; it often put me to shame that every such small gesture was so important to her.

Her consultant said all the right things and she agreed with his advice. He told her she had tried every possible treatment option and that his duty now was to ensure she was comfortable.

He believed and indicated to her that she needed more sedation to control her distressing respiratory symptoms, and he told her he would pass this on to the palliative care team. I knew she was at the end stage of her life and I am sure she did also. She gratefully acknowledged and accepted his advice and thanked him again. He waved at both of us and left the room.

Before the two families arrived that morning, we said our goodbyes with loving words and murmurings but did not utter the farewell word. Holding hands and gentle stroking and caressing was our language of love. I gave her one final kiss on the lips and after a few long moments she simply said, 'It is strange.' They were her last intimate words to me.

PART THREE

25

ONE YEAR LATER

Dear Mum,
When I start writing the book, it will be ours only for the time it takes to complete. The longer I spend at it, the more about me it will become, and so for it to work, I must also hurry. Since we are writing it together, your voice will be heard and even though I will cringe at your sentence construction, grammar and punctuation, I cannot change it and won't object, as long as I know your words will be read! For my voice to work, I cannot pick and choose but must stay honest, tell all and stop – and then it belongs to the readers.
Love, Dad

Dear Dad,
Stop all that 'mumbo-jumbo', and get on with it!
Love, Mum.

I commenced the creative writing course on memoirs in late October 2018. I was the oldest in the class and hoped to pick up some tips that would make me famous! I had no time to waste, as a literary career if it happened would be short and dependent on one offering about a remarkable woman. All my classmates wanted to write bestsellers. Towards the end of the course our teacher told us – albeit, I am convinced, with tongue in cheek – that he was so impressed with the range and breadth of our literary talents, he expected our first published works to hit the shelves in the near future. Praise is a useful form of flattery for debut authors. At the very least, I was encouraged by his enthusiasm.

One of the unusual features of the course was that before you knew it you were sharing your life story with strangers. I was struck by how spontaneous and 'therapeutic' it seemed to be, and there was nothing contrived about how it unfolded. Suddenly one becomes part of a family of kindred spirits, in a setting where outpourings of personal joys and sorrows are shared. It only takes one classmate to break the ice for a cascade of revelations to be unleashed. I tried to hide my personal loss but it came out gradually over the few months, and when I read the poem I had written about the photograph of Kathleen at Peter and Nerea's wedding in Spain, I realised they all knew already.

In early November 2018 Kathleen's sister Joan and I attended the annual Mass in Mount Anville for past pupils who had died during the year. Many of those who were there were between

50 and 80 years of age. They all looked ten years younger, as women of an age tend to do, and also because they are living healthier and subsequently longer lives. The sameness about their sense of decorum and poise on this occasion was striking, as if they had never left their alma mater – even though they were long-separated friends attending a ceremony of remembrance for deceased colleagues. This was the purpose of the gathering, but in a sense they had also come to witness and celebrate their own lives before they too passed on. It seemed as if they were in a space that had never changed, gracious to each other and proud of lives well spent and of more than modest accomplishments. Their Catholic faith was displayed with subdued respect and attention, and clearly embraced by them collectively for its continuity, common interest and humanity.

I knew the priest who was the chief celebrant and was sure there would be a good homily. But who am I to judge, and what do I mean by a 'good' homily? I suppose it is one that is carefully crafted in advance because of the occasion, and there is a palpable sense of anticipation as all the congregation sit forward to listen, as if it was about them. And so it was that day. The priest spoke to us in conversational mode about how to be like God by being human. He quoted from a number of theological experts to make his case, but he did not need to, as he was an excellent communicator and we believed him. Such a presentation strikes a chord that stays in the memory for days – a sure sign of a message successfully transmitted. It also becomes a subject for informed conversation and chat that enlivens the tea and biscuit circuits of Mass goers before they disperse to resume their separate lives again. The Mount Anville ceremony was such an event.

Before the end of Mass the names of all who had died in the past year, including Kathleen, were read out solemnly from the altar dais and were silently acknowledged. On leaving the chapel we were greeted at the door by two bowls laden with daffodil bulbs, and many of us took one or two bulbs home to plant as a symbol of our shared spiritual solidarity. After the customary tea and biscuits, Joan brought me on a tour of the school where Kathleen had been head girl in 1966, past the imposing portrait of Mater Admirabilis, still gazing down approvingly at the present pupils. The big classrooms with their high ceilings, the wide corridors, the window benches and the half-spiral staircases were still in use. We then walked outside, past the adjoining convent, before heading down a long avenue in the large school grounds to the nuns' private graveyard. I was struck by the wide-open space, the expansive vegetation and the neat hedgerows, all protecting the seat of learning from the nearby houses of the encroaching city.

The cemetery was a calm oasis laid out to order. The simple, plain headstones were small and their engraved text spare and quiet, the inscription noting only each sister's name and age. It was their remarkable longevity that made one wonder about the secret to a long and fruitful life. The vast majority lived into their 80s and beyond. Was it due to a healthy lifestyle with no smoking, no alcohol and no crème brûlée – or was it due to a stress-free work–life balance conducted within a hive of gainful activity, with an adjacent home and a garden? I was impressed by their ability to mix a busy, productive life of service with protected time and space for solitary, peaceful reflection. It confirmed to me that one can practise prayer and faith amidst all the noise of life. I promised to share this observation with my children before it was too late!

That evening I planted my two daffodil bulbs in the garden in Collon, after freeing a breathing space for them amidst the spreading ivy. I placed a wooden stake beside them to monitor their progress through winter and spring. Unbeknownst to me, Joan had planted hers on Kathleen's grave. All four bloomed undiminished throughout the spring and made merry on both terrains.

Life's journey sets you on your way with a blessing,
And puts you to rest with acclaim.

❖

It was lunchtime at the end of November 2018 in Dublin's north inner city. It was already wet and windy, and Storm Diana was on the way. I had been in the Mater library all morning working on the book. I had just bought my Christmas sambo – a constant on café menus at that time of year – and a mug of tea in Delisuz just off Blessington Street and was walking back to the education centre to eat alone. For some reason I thought about the parable of the loaves and fishes – the sambo was big enough to feed a small inner-city family! My train of thought was interrupted by a Dublin landlord standing in the entryway to a block of flats. He greeted me: 'Hello, it's a very windy day, isn't it? It's drinking weather – not a day for skirts!' I mumbled something in return and hurried on my way. I sat on a wooden bench in the small enclosed patio at the back of the education centre and ate half the sandwich before walking over to Berkeley Road Church to light three candles. When I returned to the library in the early afternoon, I opened my notebook and started composing the next chapter of the book.

The library closed at four and I went back to the church, where the organist was practising his music scores. My three candles had gone out. There were stacks of new candles waiting to be purchased and ready for more intentions. A small, select group of holy parishioners had arrived to recite the rosary and pray for the holy souls and sinners. The leader of the prayers, a tall, lean man in his early 80s, could not be heard because of the crescendo sound of the organ, and so the group packed together in a single pew. When there was a pause in the organ recital, this man raised his almighty 'Our Father Who Art in Heaven' voice. The organist understood and took his cue that it was time for prayers and that play had to stop. I felt tired then and joined in the prayers for a short while.

I had another two hours to wait before my writing class was due to start, and I decided to visit the Hugh Lane Gallery on Parnell Square, which was nearby. The alternative to prayers was to sit and listen to a recording of a TV interview in which the artist Francis Bacon described his chaos theory. It was not very conducive or inspirational to the nature of the memoir but he might take some credit for my new, more loosely structured writing style. Kathleen did not spend much time in galleries. She was always too busy for such high-brow pursuits. I reflected that I was glad I had finally written a poem for her as part of the course work for the writing class. And now, with this book, I am very pleased at the prospect that it will appear in print.

❖

It was the beginning of December 2018, and while waiting for the bus to Dublin I took shelter under the eaves of our house at the gate door. A small robin appeared on the pathway to greet me just as my mobile signalled the arrival of an email. It was from the *Irish Times*, forwarding a draft of the acknowledgement notice of Kathleen's first anniversary, which I had composed and sent the previous day. It's a custom in Ireland to formally thank people for their expressions of sympathy and attendance at funeral ceremonies by placing a notice in the national or regional newspapers on the anniversary date. Kathleen never forgot anniversaries or birthdays and always marked them with a card and often a present. It was in that manner she conducted all her relationships. She understood the importance of acknowledgement and of praise at home as well as in the workplace, where teamwork is critical to success.

I thought back to Kathleen's funeral Mass, almost a year before. My brother, the priest Teddy Lennon, had led the celebration of her life and framed his homily in the form of a conversation with her:

'You asked to have the Mass here in Navan, because this is where you spent your working life. Unlike Finbar, you loved having a crowd around you and today he is grateful they came to wish you Godspeed. When God came to call you home, your bags were packed and you were ready to go. I was listening to two women outside the church last night and one said to the other, "Now that she is gone, nothing will ever be the same again." You did some good during your time here, you made a difference and you will be remembered.'

When I arrived in Dublin, I visited Berkeley Road Church again to listen to the organ music. Again, I found myself reflecting on writing the book. Is it Kathleen and I, or Kathleen and me? It depends, but it matters. I paid my way with candles to keep her memory alive and flowing through my mind. I prayed for important random moments of recollection, though that day was not a productive one. What would Yeats think of this inspirational approach, or did he believe? Can you mix flights of mirth with faith and will it work for all the chapters and especially the dark ones to come?

❖

Uneasy feeling at the edge of control
sitting buckled in turbulence, afraid.
A sense of foreboding, transient and
stilled as control regained.

I flew to Edinburgh on 20 December 2018 and bussed to my hotel, fearing the worst. Ruth had phoned me a week earlier to tell me she was six weeks' pregnant but that her scan indicated an impending miscarriage. No heartbeat had been found and no growth of the foetus had occurred in the week since her first scan. She was anxious and upset, and in addition had very severe nausea, which I have always thought is a good sign of a viable pregnancy. She was due a definitive follow-up scan the following morning.

Finn was as chirpy as ever but had not grown since I had seen him six weeks earlier. Little wonder, as his diet on display that evening at our supper in my hotel was mainly tomato ketchup and cheese licks between small bites of chocolate biscuits! The only positive sign of nutrition was that he was drinking a reasonable quantity of milk. He reminded me of his uncle Peter, who at the same age caused Mum and me countless sleepless nights, worrying about the state of his nutrition. I had been utilising many of the same 'tricks and treats' strategies on Finn that I employed with Peter to attempt to engage productively with his upper gastrointestinal tract! Little did Kathleen and I know then how tall and handsome Peter was to become. This thought should have relieved my anxiety but I had become a worrier since Mum had died.

Ruth reassured me about Finn but my main concern that night was her. I engaged her in small talk and reassuring murmurings, and after she went home to bed, I sent her a few encouraging texts and emojis. I was unable to read or write and went to bed early. I was depending on the candles I had lit prior to my trip for a good scan result for Ruth but was not hopeful.

I spent the following morning visiting the three main libraries in Edinburgh and, after two futile forays, found the Count Tolstoy book in the National Library – I wanted to do a little research about his connection to Greenlawns. Just before I had completed the paperwork to access the reading room, I had a good-news call from Ruth to tell me they had found a heartbeat and that the pregnancy was intact. The candles worked on this occasion! I vowed once more to re-evaluate my faith and beliefs and to be less critical of my Catholic upbringing. I bought a cappuccino in the canteen and sat down to read the magazine of the National Library of Scotland. As I gazed at the wandering crowd in the nearby reading room, I penned a poem on its back cover:

It is nearly noon and most of my companion souls
are silent women passing time.
The featured artists were all household names,

and yet it was as if I had just discovered them
in my latter years, and can only choose one more
to study before I fade away.
I cherished the interlude, dreaming
of the elevated station I briefly ruled.

On my way back to Ruth's apartment I went into Blackwell's bookstore; browsing through the Classics section, I came across Leo Tolstoy's novella, *The Death of Ivan Ilyich*. A few weeks later I read it on one of my bus trips to and from Dublin. It was short enough to read in one sitting. The book recounts the progression of the fatal illness of the title character, and is said to have been inspired by the real-life story of an individual living near Tolstoy's home in Tula, who died of 'stomach cancer' in 1881. I read it again one week later and was intrigued by its description of Ilyich's illness and the many parallels with Kathleen's presentation. The main character in the book, Ivan Ilyich, is a judge and thus in a similar station in life to Kathleen. Tolstoy's description of Ilyich's illness fits more with a diagnosis of pancreatic cancer than stomach cancer; either of these could have been the primary source of Kathleen's cancer. Pancreatic cancer is still very difficult to diagnose at an early stage, and even today is often only identified when it has spread. Ilyich's doctors do not know what is wrong with him either at the beginning or the end. They think it is a benign illness at first and only much later on do they acknowledge it is likely to be of a more serious nature, though they remain baffled about its cause: 'The doctors could not decide. Well, they could, but they all decided differently.' This is not a reason in itself for criticism as in Kathleen's case the source of her cancer was never found, but the nature and gravity of her illness was established at the outset.

Ilyich's presenting complaint is left flank pain which he becomes aware of after a minor fall. It does not bother him at first and does not interfere with his work or lifestyle. When it becomes increasingly severe and constant, his wife urges him to see a doctor. At this stage he is worried that something is seriously wrong and needs empathy and reassurance. He does not get either in a consultation with his doctor and leaves the surgery confused and angry. As time goes by, it is clear that he is fading away and that the clinical signs of cancer are evident to himself, his family and friends. Second opinions from self-styled experts are unhelpful. As a patient he is angry at the helplessness of the doctors, but most of all at their lack of compassion and his belief that they are withholding information from him about his illness. In the 1880s very little was known about cancer, so Ilyich's doctors could not have diagnosed what was wrong with him anyway. At the end stage of his illness, they have to resort to overdosing him with opioids to hasten his departure.

One of Kathleen's presenting complaints was also left flank pain, which she initially thought was musculoskeletal in origin and I had no clinical reason to believe otherwise. Fortunately for us, however, her treatment at the hands of the medical profession could not have been more different from that of Ilyich. From the outset, her doctors realised how important empathy and reassurance were to her care plan. Her pain was a constant concern but she was able to cope with it, knowing that they were near at hand and ready to assist her in any way they could.

However, even now, more than a century later, some particular cancers continue to baffle doctors and have yet to reveal all their secrets, and treatment in such cases is a combination of symptomatic and palliative care. In my head I know that remarkable progress has been achieved in making cancer a manageable long-term disease for many people today; and even in Kathleen's case, I am grateful that her oncologist did his best to ensure that during the short extension she was afforded, her quality of life was good. My heart however aches that the particular lot she drew did not allow her a fighting chance for more time.

26

A MIDWINTER GARDEN, THE ROBIN AND THE CANDLES

The first winter without Kathleen was bittersweet. During those long bleak months, I would often go outside and sit on the old garden bench and see the same robin perching on a nearby chair or flitting about the lawn in front of me. Of course, the robin didn't know Kathleen was gone and was likely to be one of many that had spent time in the garden with us over recent years, unconcerned about our presence and proximity but acting out the role of a companion anyway. I'd gaze forlornly at my mobile phone, which was now largely silent, and realise I didn't have anybody to call or text on a whim anymore, as most of those communications would have been to Kathleen. I was never a fan of 'the mobile'. It was a nuisance to me and I never became dependent on it, whereas to her it was essential for work and for family life. She had over 600 contacts in her phone, whereas I had less than 30.

Sitting there in the garden, I would sometimes briefly consider making contact with a close friend but then realise that I would normally only do so for a specific purpose, and that to increase the frequency of contact now would feel contrived, and might also invite unwanted attention. And so I desisted. I'd feel ashamed and selfish for indulging myself and hear Kathleen admonishing me and urging me to get on with the book and with my life.

That first year, I had to work twice as hard in the garden to maintain its craggy beauty. When all the leaves fall and the winter sets in, the year's work comes to nought again. The heavy, sodden logs of wood that once were branches lie beside the stone walls, begging to be removed from the nearby trees that nurtured them. The grass plots are now a carpet of brown slippery mush covered with brittle twigs spread by the winter winds. For a while it is desolate, and days and even weeks might go by without a garden visit or even a walk along the wet leaf-filled paths to breathe in the cold air. Where does the energy come from to take up the burden anew? It comes from the birds, the ramrod daffodil stalks and the peeping snowdrops. For the first year it was an act of remembrance, a duty fulfilled – but without her, can it be sustained?

As I finished my breakfast on New Year's Eve 2018, I glanced out the kitchen window and saw the first snowdrops at the foot of the holly tree and had a quiet weep. Then I reached out and put my morning pills into my mouth, just as another pang of loss struck. I felt a sudden choking sensation as I leapt to my feet to cough and splutter, and my respiratory distress resolved in seconds. Self-pity is not good for my health, it seems! At the time I was acutely aware there was nobody about to thump my back and release the foreign body from my windpipe. Where were you, Heimlich, when I needed you? I had only recently been reading a study from Rice University in Houston, which said that the surviving spouse or partner is at increased risk of dying of heart disease within six months of being bereaved. I had only just escaped that fate and missed being the subject of a case report on a patient choking to death from a broken heart!

On the morning of Kathleen's first anniversary, I saw the robin again, perched on the bonnet of my car as I was about to bring my grandson for a walk. I was greatly preoccupied with the task of finishing the book, and by this time, I reckoned I was more than halfway there. Kathleen was right that, whenever I'm giving a speech or some other kind of public address, I tend to go on and on. For me, it is more to do with ensuring the penny drops, but I suppose often it does not, and the audience stops listening to me. On the other hand, my writing is much more precise and exact and the message is always clear, sometimes jarringly clear. I wanted the book to make up for my deficiencies as an orator and make Kathleen proud that I have struck the right notes and tone this time. I had been pleased with the feedback on my writing skills and the positive response to my style of delivery at the most recent creative writing session. While I had read a lot of memoirs in the previous year, none had any great defining influence on my approach. The most important part of a book is the ending. The beginning is easy. The middle part is the most difficult to write. I could see the truth of that now. I was trying to tell a personal story that was in many senses over, at the same time as I was having to move forward in the present world. Kathleen's story had ended a year ago, but I had been able to stay in her zone with the aid of the robin, the candles and the garden.

The Catholic faith is alive and well in Navan, and for her Anniversary Mass, the faithful were out in force. A perceptive address by the parish priest added to the ceremony. I was gratified to see that some notice had been taken of my previous representations to the effect that more attention should be given to other feast days in the Church's calendar; that, for example, that day's Epiphany deserves more exposure and that the dependence on Christmas and Easter should be tempered. Though both of these are, of course, the alpha and omega of the Christian faith, it is important to maintain the devotional spirit throughout the religious cycle.

After the Anniversary Mass, Kathleen's courage and qualities of character were recounted and affirmed again to me by her siblings. 'Moving on swiftly and not dwelling on the bad stuff – that was her mantra.' 'She managed our parents through their old age with a gentleness and respect that allowed them to end their days in a most dignified manner.' 'Her focus was absolute, on any task or project she took on.' 'When she took up painting in her final months, she did not need instruction. She was a natural and, just like everything she undertook, she excelled at it.' Later that evening, as those who had stayed on after the Mass were leaving to go their separate ways, a lady who had known Kathleen very well came up to me and asked how I was getting on. I told her it had been a difficult year but that I was coping, and thanked her. She wished me well and then, as she took her leave, she said, 'You do know, of course, that the second year is worse.'

Meanwhile, the acknowledgement notice in the *Irish Times* had been seen by a number of her colleagues, who texted during the day to wish me well. That night, as I was getting ready for bed, while looking through some old correspondence I came across a comment about Kathleen's mother in a reference she had received in 1944 from a professor in her alma mater in Galway, where he commented that 'her personality weighs in her favour'. I reflected that it was an observation that equally applied to her eldest daughter.

The next day, I went to Mass in Collon, where Kathleen's anniversary was also acknowledged. On the way into the church, I noted that there was a collection for St Vincent de Paul, then a church door collection, followed by two further ones during Mass: one for the parish and another for the priests. I am not sure the faithful can afford such multiple calls on their modest incomes. The faith will not survive such constant 'holy requests'. The local community's acknowledgement of her memory was graciously communicated to me with glances, head nods and handshakes.

❖

I met Jimmy, a patient in the Mater, in mid-January 2019, when he agreed to participate in my bedside tutorial. Normally the tutor picks the patients for me and sends me the names the evening before, but on this occasion he was away on leave and I had to find a few suitable cases myself on the morning of the class. I came across Jimmy by chance and took a brief history from him. He was comfortable, alert and in good form but worried about his predicament, which he explained to me. He had an advanced bowel cancer that was first diagnosed in 2016. It was one of the more common cancers. He had undergone multiple surgeries and had two courses of chemotherapy, which, he said, 'knocked the living daylights out of me'. All his treatment options had been exhausted and a palliative intervention – a stent placement – to relieve a high small-bowel obstruction had failed. His doctor had just told him that the plan now was to discharge him home to the palliative care team or, in Jimmy's words, 'home to die'.

At this point, Jimmy became emotional, and I asked him where he was from.

'I am from Navan, and I used to work in the hospital,' he replied.

'You probably knew my wife, Dr McGarry?'

'Of course I did. She was a great doctor.'

I told him about her Anniversary Mass, which had taken place the previous week.

'Yes, I knew about it from the parish bulletin,' he said. Jimmy was the same age as Kathleen and was first diagnosed about the same time. The natural history of his disease was similar and it was certain the outcome would be the same. When I left his room, I became emotional too. After the tutorial, I met Jimmy's wife briefly, and she told me he was due to be discharged back to the hospital in Navan the next day. Before I left the ward that morning, I called in again to see him and told him I would visit him when he was transferred.

Ten days later I dropped in to the hospital in Navan. I asked the receptionist, who knew me, what ward Jimmy was in, and she replied, 'Did you not know? He was buried yesterday.' Before leaving again, I decided to stop off at the hospital chapel. I knew a reflective citation about Kathleen's contribution to the hospital, written by one of her colleagues, had been on display there for four months. I had a WhatsApp picture of it on my phone, but I had not read it or been to see it in the hospital. It was hanging outside the chapel and there was nobody about. As I read it, with her photograph affixed alongside, I became tearful again. I managed to leave unnoticed, thinking of her and of Jimmy. On reaching my car, I thought of Ruth and counted my blessings that her pregnancy was back on track.

❖

On the first weekend in March 2019, Ruth came home from Edinburgh and Joan came up to Collon to sort out Mum's wardrobes. They found six in four separate rooms, all packed with clothes. Some had remained there for years, undisturbed by any hands other than Kathleen's; in the two most out-of-the-way wardrobes, a light layer of dust had evenly accumulated on the cuffs and sleeves of the coats and dresses, meaning that even she had not moved them for some time.

While this painful and sensitive 'spring cleaning' was being undertaken, I was dispatched outdoors, but not before Joan did a garden inspection with me. Everything was overgrown and unkempt and needed immediate attention if the plants were to bloom again. My big problem had always been with Mum's favourite hydrangeas, which suffered frequent injury and decay under my watch. Even now that she is gone, I am afraid to go near some of the plants and flowers with a cutting tool because somewhere up there she is watching over me! But by this time, I was no longer afraid of the hydrangeas. This was partly because I knew that, no matter how much injury I caused, they would bloom again. If I could not be reckless here and scream quietly in rough-hewn language, what was the point of it all?

After Joan's short lesson, I set about my garden work while the serious labour was conducted indoors. Weeding was my favourite pastime, and when my back began to ache that day, I changed posture and moved around on bended knee to complete the task. The closer I got to the grass, the more weeds I saw — and when I went down on both knees, they were everywhere! Next for attention was the ivy, which needed clearing — another source of pleasure for a surgeon. Extracting the carpet of ground ivy required long arm sweeps as I crawled with purpose across the soil with accompanying secateurs. Then, after removing my industrial gloves, I began with bare fingers to pluck its spreading tentacles from the walls and tree trunks. When I stood back and surveyed my work, I experienced the same sense of achievement I used to feel after performing a difficult surgical operation. The garden was a safe place to plunder and unleash my repressed emotions without fear of harm.

By the end of the weekend the garden was recovering, and the multiple black bin bags were full of Mum's clothes and ready for delivery to the St Vincent de Paul charity shops. There was much more work to be done in the garden and the wardrobes, and it was clear that both tasks would require ongoing dedication and labour for some time to come. I know now I won't live forever and will not take the garden with me or the clothes or the poems. I can die without the latter two — but I will miss the garden.

In the manner Kathleen used to weigh up the pluses …

Good things: she was not forgotten; her patients continued to talk fondly about her; the two grandchildren were well and were growing up; Ruth had taken on the baton of 'parent minder' and contacted me every day; the robin was a regular visitor and I had started the yearly garden work cycle again; I was writing again and hoped to have the first draft of the book completed within a matter of months.

EPILOGUE

To touch the soil on bended knee,
To flake the gravel free of grass,
To pluck the weeds along the path,
To break the twigs to fill the sack,
To pour the jugs to wet the plants.
To walk the shore to hear the waves,
To light the wick to call the saints,
To live alone to feel the loss,
To write the words to tell the tale.

It was St Patrick's Day 2019 and I had now exhausted my 'creative writing talents' and completed the first draft, and so it was time to close the first chapter in the book's production. It had been a labour of love and filled most of the time since Kathleen had died. Her memory was alive and beside me in the study and garden, and I did not need any other social sustenance apart from my friend Jeremy and the medical students. They were important too. I was not sure I could manage but had decided to resume my tutorials in the Mater a few weeks after she died. On my own at home in winter, I found it difficult to cope with the isolation, and so a bus ride up and down to Dublin passed most of a day. The students knew nothing about Kathleen, and my interaction with them was as before. I did, however, have to watch out for medical colleagues and used to scan the footpaths and hospital corridors to see if anybody I knew was approaching, so that I could take diversionary action. Whenever I bumped into any of them, they would try to 'break bread' but could not find the words to relieve the hunger and relied instead on asking questions about things that did not matter to me. I did not want to linger with them in the silence but to quickly move on. At that time, I was simply not ready to talk. Maybe I was expecting too much too soon.

I was lucky to have a faithful walking companion in Jeremy, who never asked questions because he already knew all the answers. During our weekly constitutional, he talked effortlessly about a potpourri of UK politics, the state of Greece, the decline of Barclays Bank since his retirement and his fascination with model railway bogies. It all amounted to good medicine for me. Aisling and Catherine from the palliative care team in Drogheda, who had been so kind and supportive to both of us, offered to meet me, presumably to check I was coping with my loss and ensure I was well. The local health service sent me a circular, offering counselling services and an invitation to a grieving course. I was not interested in either offer at the time because I did not want to grieve for her. If you grieve for somebody, they cannot come back and talk to you; the relationship is over. I wanted to hold on to her, not forget her.

Although the first draft was now completed, I soon discovered that my work on the book was by no means over. The original master copy never survived the day. As soon as I opened the desktop again, I immediately saw the errors and the strange voices jumping out at me from the screen and began the next revision. And the same thing happened again, many times, over the months that followed. Angela, the librarian in the Mater education centre library, would kindly print out each new draft I penned, and when I got home, I'd place the pages on the top shelf in the study. Their life span was short as new printouts replaced them in no time.

I knew that finding a publisher was my next logical step and was ready for the rejections I'd been told would inevitably follow. When you receive rejection letters, it is reasonable to assume somebody from the publishing house has read your proposal, and that in itself is a positive. As we'd been told in the writing class, a rejection is best regarded as a starting point on your literary journey and not a final judgement on your work. And it is infinitely better than receiving no acknowledgement at all, which had been my experience with a publisher during the previous summer. Six weeks after sending in my proposal, I phoned its office and was told the material had been received and advised that it might take some more time to receive a response. 'Well, you are going to miss a trick,' I was minded to say, but contained myself. When I still hadn't heard anything six months later, I admitted defeat and realised I had set the bar too high. After reading my covering letter again, I concluded that the first and last sentences were critical and that I might have slipped up. 'I have never written a book and use pen and paper for all my first drafts' was my opening line, and after 1,000 intervening words of passion, human interest and seduction, my last sentence concluded with – 'This is a shot in the dark but aiming high is always worthwhile'! Around the same time, I sent an early partial draft to a Jesuit friend and to a world-acclaimed literary critic, and received two nuanced acknowledgements that I was able to decipher as words of encouragement. That was enough to go back to the well – and I resolved that I wouldn't show it to anyone else until I had completed a full revised draft.

It was a wet wintery evening in April 2019 in Dublin and I had arranged to meet my eldest son, a junior barrister, for an early-bird supper before accompanying him to a book launch in the law chambers. I wanted to see how such an event is staged. I was already sodden from the rain and did not stay long. I bought a signed copy of the book (which I would subsequently lose on my way home), but as I was leaving the hall, I paused to listen to the editorial director of the publishing house, who was speaking on stage about the book. I forgot her name but something about her stuck in the memory. A month later, my youngest son helped me find her on LinkedIn, and with his help I sent a message to her which she picked up. My pitch to her was that I was also from King's County and I was looking for a publisher for a very special memoir. She invited me to send a few chapters to her and said she was impressed with the author's voice.

Serendipity has been a companion all my life. I am very much aware that the road to finding a publisher can be a very long, difficult and frustrating one. The publishing industry is not always the writer's friend and the author's voice alone is often not enough to gain favour. I was impressed by the work of my classmates on the creative writing course: each had a variety of voices in their work and many had travelled through the literary maze in order to discover their best moves. Writers forge their paths in different ways, and the course was a good springboard for me. When it comes to getting published, strong writing and perseverance are key, but good luck has also a very important part to play. I know how fortunate I have been that things fell into place for me.

❖

I returned to our holiday home in Connemara recently to unwind, reflect and refresh my memories of Kathleen in the place where we spent our happiest times together with our children and each other.

At rest on the edge among rocks,
gazing at the flat ocean quietly lapping
at the nearby clad of seaweed.
The sound of smothered thunder
was just a distant plane.
The sky was blue above
but white and grey clouds
were filling from the west.
The grey clouds break and spread,
but hold their load.
The gentle breeze is warm.
The few minutes passed alone, but longer
than the normal din and free of posture.
A break for breath and au revoir.

Connemara was the place of her leave-taking; a comfort zone beside the ocean, where time and space stand still. The sounds and motions of the sea can be heard and seen from our holiday house just above the pier. It was here she enjoyed the simple pleasures of the season: reading, walking and seeking shelter from the wind and rain. This was where she braved the sea with her short and deliberate swimming forays, conducted out of reach of the water sprays of encouragement generated by me to get her down and under the waves. She was happier paddling on Lettergesh and Glassilaun beaches, with me beside her on a parallel track on dry sand, and joining up at regular intervals for a kiss and cuddle out of sight of other eyes. It was here also where our communal boat, the precious *Rib*, under the command of our own commodore held the swells at bay while we gazed in awe at Turk and Bofin with our summer friends. We told tall tales of many mighty men unperched since last time, reputations scalded and discarded before we docked for lunch. Over the holiday stay, similar opportunities to enhance and diminish reputations were indulged in before supper on dry land. The daily routine did not vary unless we chose to break the spell.

Connemara is a place where past memories endure because the landscape never changes, and for me that weekend was a visit of renewal. It was quiet and serene, its beauty undiminished and its welcome low-key but real. I was accompanied by my sister Maev. We called by Bridie, Margaret and the two Johns to share good wishes and honour long friendships and to collect the keys of Silverstrand. After unloading the car we set about retracing the familiar walks in cold, wintery conditions of intermittent strong winds, rain and short dry spells.

The next morning, we met the retired local community nurse on the hillside, who sympathised with me on my loss. We stopped for a rest break in the Renvyle House Hotel and met Ronnie, the general manager, who welcomed me back with complimentary coffee and biscuits. Renvyle House was once the home of my alter ego, St John Gogarty. He bought it in 1917 and made it his bolt hole in the west, where he spent many long, relaxing weekends entertaining his literary friends. The place is still full of Gogarty memorabilia. On our way out we passed the outdoor pool where all our children learned to swim. We continued the loop walk on the roadside back to Tully, past the Teach Ceoil and then back to Silverstrand. Maev checked her Fitbit to confirm that the 12,000-steps mark had been passed. Tullymore Danny and Oisín, the two Connemara ponies that seemed to spend their lives in the field beside the ocean, were nowhere to be seen that day. Finn would have been disappointed!

After Mass in Tullycross next morning, I thanked the young pianist (a local schoolteacher) and the choir and complimented them on the communion reflection hymn, 'How Can I Repay the Lord?' As I was leaving, I looked up and marvelled again at Harry Clarke's stained-glass window depiction of Saints Bernard and Barbara with Christ revealing his Sacred Heart. I had a sudden pang of regret, as my weekly visit to Kathleen's grave was overdue and I worried that she had missed me. In bed that evening I was unsettled and recalled Donald Hall's 'Midwinter Letter' to his dead wife. Now I also sadly appreciate that same agony that strikes me when I remember both the good and the bad times.

I visit her grave at least once a week. It is a little over an hour's drive from Collon, in a quiet landscaped park in a valley below the Dublin mountains. Her inscribed name and time on earth is all the headstone reveals and is a focus for eye contact. It invites greeting and an exchange of words, a reaffirmation of humanity.

Since her death I have never stopped talking to her. I give her all the week's news and the mundane tittle-tattle she sought from me in life. On my last visit I heard her voice.

'Dad, have you told everyone I am dead? I am still getting emails from the medical locum agencies seeking my services to cover annual leave for colleagues in Navan and Sligo. I also get regular requests from my college inquiring about my availability to participate in the Membership examination and receive circulars from my professional representative organisation to advise me on how to apply for back-pay due to me!'

And so I responded to her: 'I am not surprised, Mum, I am still being sent your eFlow and electricity bills, and despite my calls and emails to inform them you are no longer in a position to pay, they persist with their customary practice. I suppose as long as the bills are paid, they don't mind!'

That response seemed to satisfy her as she did not say anymore. I then said my usual prayer, had a quiet weep and wished her well until next time.

You cannot prepare for loss. Even when it happens or months later, it takes time to feel it. Only when you have picked up the pieces and put them away somewhere does it strike. You then wake up one morning with nothing more to do. No one else can fill the void. No one moves, talks, smiles or laughs the same. All the familiar spaces are empty, and the cawing birds and passing cars are louder than before. The noise leans on the closed door as the day becomes longer, no matter the season, no more determined by light and darkness.

Her stoical nature and my emotional gene were always part of our working dynamic and are still in play now. Because I loved her, I want her goodness and kindness to last and for the people who knew her to remember her. I now have to learn to live without her. During her illness we both had to awaken and renew our faith. First we had to find it. For that, we needed time and it came, spare and in abundance. We found the way ahead separately and together, and I am sure her faith sustained her throughout her illness when all else was falling by the wayside. There was no succour in knowledge but there is consolation in remembrance and, despite the distance and after 50 years, I am not gone from her, or she from me.

This poem was also written 50 years ago, probably for myself, but is not as inane as some of its peers. It is still a dreadful rendition of the art of poetry but perhaps now is prescient in that it contains some elements of the untainted faith and spirit of the time of my upbringing that I have managed to retain in spite of everything.

When I want to fly
I climb and wave my arms,

and close my lips and blow
and scatter all the wind,
and hop on single feet from grass to stone,
and whiff and smell and shake my hair,
and laugh and breathe the air,
and scream and shout and cry,
and no one gives a damn
'cause I'm alone and free.
And when I want to land,
to come back home,
to bricks and crowds, to shops
to fumes and stuffy men who sweat,
I pause and lift my arms again
and look back up and see the blue,
Just blue and Heaven – it is all blue,
and cry a little more,
and flap my wings and shout anew –
The Heavens are all blue.

So, it is you,
And you will call
When I call,
And do what I do.

She did not plan this ending. It's funny how most people go
into hospital to get better. Kathleen was fighting the disease and

the treatment, and her only chance was to stay out of hospital. Everyone knows they are going to die and most never give it a second thought. It becomes scary if you know when and how it is going to happen, which she did. Her temporal life was one of ambition, courage and more than modest accomplishment, but at the end of the day just a footprint in the sand, washed away in an instant by the incoming tide. Her soul, however, survives and lies somewhere in the pages of this book.

ACKNOWLEDGEMENTS

Do not scan down. You will not see your name. It is a short list and leaves out many deserving of mention. I am grateful to my brother and sisters, and to Kathleen's brothers and sisters, who have stayed by my shoulder, the next-door neighbours who have kept in touch, the friends who phone from time to time, the colleagues who still remember her, the workmates in Navan who tell me they miss her.

I thank my classmates and the master on the creative writing course for helping me find my voice, the wise and gifted Jesuit who encouraged me and the acclaimed literary critic who did not demur. I also thank the young Irish author who told me to focus on the garden.

I acknowledge my good fortune and delight that the senior editor discovered me and the working editor turned a surgeon into an author.

Finally I salute Kathleen, the love of my life, for her foresight and courage in commencing this project of discovery and I hope she will be proud and happy with the outcome.

PERMISSION ACKNOWLEDGEMENTS